To the cancer patient

For those who are confronted with cancer or who loves someone who is, this is a book written for you.

It is a direct and factual look at the path through discovery, diagnosis, treatment, and recovery, presented in understandable language with frank information about the journey about to be taken.

Catharine Scott writes of her experience with an irrepressible sense of hope and her joy of life.

In the words of the author, "This book contains the type of information I wish had been available to me."

All who enter this daunting and challenging world can learn from one who has made the journey, and who has brought this information out for you.

ONLY
IF YOU
REALLY
WANT
TO KNOW

Breast Cancer
Coping Hints
and Treatment Side Effects

By Catharine Bracken Scott

With Nancy Bracken Fuller

Only if You Really Want to Know
by
Catharine Bracken Scott

Published by

Therapeia Biblion, an imprint of
Fountain City Publishing Company
P.O. Box 18477
Knoxville, TN   37928
orders at:
        www.FCPub.com/Therapeia

DISCLAIMER

Any product names used in this book are meant as examples only, and solely as a suggestion of product type based on the author's personal experiences in dealing with her cancer experience. Proper names used in this book are not meant in any way to be an exclusive endorsement of a particular brand, institution, or medical professional, nor to deny endorsement of competitor brands, products, or services.

The author does not claim legal affiliation with any organization mentioned in these pages. In some anecdotal cases fictional names have been substituted for actual names of people.

In all cases, advice of your physician should be given priority over any suggestions in this book. This is not a medical book. The primary goal of this book is to help ease the suffering and discomfort of those who face the challenge of cancer, and to help the family members and friends who support her in her trials.

Web sites and phone numbers in this book are current as of publication
        -Editor

Copyright © 2006

Print First Edition ISBN 13: 978-0-9760867-1-0
Print First Edition ISBN 10: 0-9760867-1-9

Library of Congress Control Number: 2006924275

First Printing August 2006

Dear Breast Cancer Patients,

This book contains the type of information I wish had been available to me after my own diagnosis and during my subsequent breast cancer treatment. My true purpose for writing it is to bring you comfort and hope by including some suggestions I was unable to find elsewhere. The sequence of each chapter is based on my personal schedule. This is also true regarding the information and interpretations contained herein. Although your cancer experience may be quite different from mine, hopefully our therapy will be similar enough for you to feel better equipped to cope with your own program by knowing what to expect.

It may be an acceptable choice for you to be unconcerned about procedures ahead of time; however, knowing what to anticipate seems to help many people cope more readily. If your choice is to prepare yourself for the worst while hoping and praying for the best, you are holding an instrument designed to enlighten and encourage you along your way toward recovery.

The internet, plus pamphlets provided by the American Cancer Society, National Cancer Institute, and other helpful groups have much free in-depth material to offer. I think you'll find this presentation somewhat more readable. I offer you some hints and sources, along with a spoonful of light humor and a sincere desire to inspire you as you fight to win this battle.

Your treatment as a patient most likely will be highly individualized by your oncologists. Remember that your reactions may vary drastically from those of mine or any other person. In your own way, you will learn how to handle whatever comes. It isn't easy to make light comments about such a heavy subject as cancer, but a positive attitude is vital.

My goal, indeed my mission, is to give you some general information about cancer, a few tips that may help you deal with possible side effects, and the absolute assurance that far more people than you can imagine are continually hoping and praying for you.

CBS

FOREWORD

by Nancy M. Copple
Supporter and Friend of Author

Cancer patients who receive this book should definitely consider themselves blessed. I can almost hear you readers say, "The woman writing this foreword must be crazy because I have been diagnosed with cancer; I'm scared and feel *cursed*, not *blessed*. I'm sure Nancy Copple has never been told that *she* has cancer."

Well, you are correct that I myself have never had to face this disease; but trust me, after reading what this author has written with all the observations and suggestions she has compiled for *you*, I know it would be the first book I would want available for *me* in that situation.

Catharine's first-hand experience with this ordeal, from diagnosis to treatments and aftermath, has enabled her to share in a realistic and caring way with all of you just what she has learned along the way.

She writes with warmth, knowledge, encouragement, hope, and yes, humor, reaching out to help others and their loved ones as they face their individual futures dealing with breast cancer.

Yes, dear reader, you are *blessed*. Read on!

DEDICATION

This book is dedicated to *you*, the doctors, nurses, and caregivers who restore health and who strive to keep hope alive in breast cancer patients, and also to those very same patients who, having faith and hope, reach out with comfort to others who need *their* support.

Our world is a better place for all who in various ways reduce the mental, physical, and spiritual suffering of other people.

THE LOGO AND ITS MEANING

My logo and its meaning signify the positive influences we each can have on the attitudes of other breast cancer patients. I call my motto REACH. As women, we strive to nurture, inspire, and uplift everyone, especially those who need and love us and those who are loved by us.

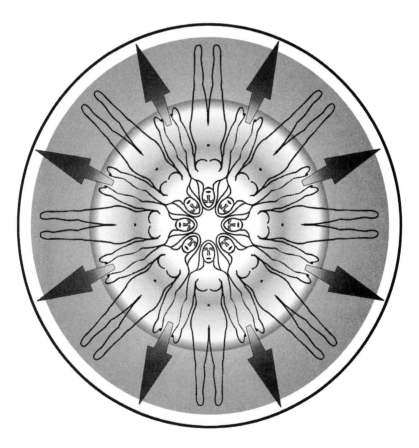

This round stained glass window design represents the earth. Its nucleus represents our inner spirit. The dark shooting arrows emanating from the center spread hope to all, but especially to the human figures which epitomize all women undergoing cancer treatment. Try to envision them like Leonardo Da Vinci's famous drawing of "The Vitruvian Man."

These women are symbolic of our own reaching as we stretch our arms *upward* to God in thanksgiving and hope for the continuing gift of life; *outward* to others with gratitude for their support; and compassionately *downward* by bending to aid all who might need encouragement. Our hopes and fears, beliefs and yearnings, our very souls are encoded and expressed through these postures of praise, love, and service. This motto is one you may have already chosen or now choose to adopt. As long as there is breath, there is time to make a difference.

Catharine Bracken Scott

TABLE OF CONTENTS

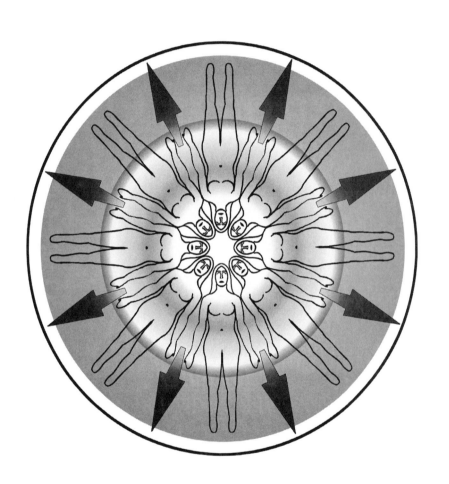

Chapter 1

Journal

ALL MEDICAL HISTORY

Record your medical history! You will find that keeping a personal journal is a great way to do that. Such data will help you recall the dates of all treatments and their side effects. You also will have a record of your feelings and when medical events occurred. This information ultimately will be essential for your own reference.

CLUE TO THE PRESENT

You may be repeatedly called upon by various doctors to remember medical information, so never withhold anything from them, no matter how embarrassing it may be for you to admit something. Doctors have heard nearly everything. Often the past becomes a clue to the present and the future when history is available to specialists.

COPING HINTS

Daily journal writing gives you an idea of what to expect on certain days after each treatment. Be sure to write down any helpful coping hints that you may pass on to others. Your journal will also remind you of your supporters and how much they do for you.

COVERAGE

Regardless of the insurance coverage you may have, some expenses will not be accepted. Many of your medical costs might be allowable deductions. Try to keep all pertinent receipts for tolls, gasoline, special clothing, etc., in the event such proof may become necessary.

KIND OF THERAPY

Even if you feel that you are not a writer, you will find that journal therapy is beneficial. Get your main thoughts and feelings down on paper without worrying about writing in "English class" style. You'll probably find that it is cathartic. Anyway, this kind of therapy is certainly less stressful than any other that you may now be enduring.

METHOD OF SELF EXPRESSION

Jotting down your thoughts and activities is important. It gives you a method of expressing what you are going through without being boring company for others, who frankly can be sympathetic and interested for only short periods of time. They just can't imagine what you are experiencing and don't want to hear too many details. Some of them are already frightened as they internalize your pains and begin to wonder if they too may have to face cancer, but most people will listen. Those who love you know it is important for you to express yourself. Your journal will serve as a sounding board for things you may not care to share verbally with others.

POST TREATMENTS

When all of your treatments are completed, you may consider making a separate list of the dates of each session, your doctors' names with phone numbers and addresses, plus your medications with dosage amounts. You'll probably need to refer to it from time to time.

STICKER SUGGESTIONS

If someone wants to do something nice for you, suggest that they may find some small blank labels. By writing key words on the stickers and placing them on the appropriate journal pages, you can more quickly locate important events. This includes information such as the dates of your surgery, various appointments, each chemotherapy and radiation session, CBC treatments, and even your nurses' names. In this way, you will become less frustrated

in seeking information that eventually you may want
or need for reference.

TODAY __/__/__

Your personal journal begins when you acquire
one of the many available books with spiral bindings
and blank pages. Then begin writing *your* story. Be
sure to date each entry.

Chapter 2

Diagnosis

DETECTION — EARLY

It is extremely important to detect any sign of breast cancer as early as possible, before the cells duplicate and spread to the lymph nodes. Your chance of survival triples if your lymph nodes are cancer-free. Knowing that certainly is worth seeing your doctor for regular check-ups!

DISCOVERY OF LUMP

If you discover a lump in your breast, go directly to your gynecologist or an oncologist. Either of them will probably return an earlier diagnosis than a general practitioner could. If a biopsy is sent to a laboratory, the pathologist is more likely to give it a higher priority.

INSURANCE

Shortly after your diagnosis, be sure to check with your insurance company regarding your financial obligations as well as theirs.

If you are too young for Medicare and unfortunate enough (for whatever reason) to be without insurance, you must turn into a detective and seek help as soon as possible. Don't allow cancer to spread because you postponed finding a way to pay for prompt care. Cancer cells multiply much too rapidly for you to procrastinate even one day.

MANY REACTIONS

When women are diagnosed, each one may react differently. Some are frightened that they will die much too soon, although in these days that is most unlikely. Many are simply angry about the disease itself and feel that they are just too busy to have to deal with it. Others are in denial, but gradually reality sets in. Some immediately accept the diagnosis and are eager to begin and win the battle. Still others cry and wonder, "Why me?" Many are quite surprised since they have been healthy all their lives and are unaware of any relatives who have had cancer. Eventually, all have to deal with the real truth of their mortality. Living a life of acceptance and a resolution to enjoy a quality existence becomes the goal of most cancer participants.

PAIN TOLERANCE

People who feel they have a zero tolerance for pain may contemplate refusing any further cancer treatment beyond surgery. Caregivers should strongly encourage these individuals to rethink their refusal inclinations. Once women realize that they will be given pain relievers, they will likely reconsider and learn to tolerate the treatments.

QUESTIONS

Second Opinion: If you have any doubts that there might be a mistake in your diagnosis or treatment, go to another doctor or hospital for a second opinion. Check with your insurance company to see if they will finance an alternate opinion; but regardless of their answer, follow through if you have any misgivings. Also, people need to be told what options they have regarding treatment and the "worst possible" as well as the "best potential" outcome to expect. If the diagnosis returned from a pathologist is inconclusive, once again, don't hesitate to suggest that your physician might use another laboratory to obtain a second diagnosis. Pathologists with different techniques may detect the cause of your problem more readily.

Timing of Pathology Report: By asking your doctor how long before the pathology report is generally returned, you won't feel stressed if it isn't done as rapidly as other tests that have been returned quickly. Sometimes pathologists need two or three days and other times it may take them a full week.

REJECTION VS. ACCEPTANCE

There is a distinct difference between denial and acceptance of one's cancer diagnosis. If you are in denial, you will gradually face the reality and the need for medical assistance to combat the illness. If you are into acceptance right away, convincing your family of that may be a rather difficult job.

RISKS OF BREAST CANCER

The chance of developing cancer is highest for women having any one of the following:

+ Personal history of cancer.
+ Mother, sister, or daughter who has had breast cancer.
+ History of breast disease, even if biopsy is proven benign.
+ *Not* having given birth before turning 30 years old.

TREATING POSSIBLE UNDETECTED CANCER CELLS

Some people opt initially to have surgery only, thereby forgoing the trauma of chemotherapy and radiation. If your oncologist suggests treating you with all three, it may be wise to agree unless you prefer to seek a second opinion first. Statistics in favor of treatments are from a 35% chance of no recurrence beyond surgery to an 80% or higher chance with treatments. Most women decide in favor of the better odds. Life is certainly worth the extra effort for additional years of good health.

Chapter 3

Surgery

BEFORE SURGERY

Anxiety: Sharing thoughts of your prognosis and upcoming surgery with fellow patients may take away much of the fear and anxiety you are bound to have. "Misery loves company" develops a whole new *positive* meaning when people become friends and confide in each other with mutual understanding.

Early Therapy: some procedures might be given prior to surgery in order to shrink the tumor. This would cause you to be stronger by building up your immune system.

Forget: Thank heaven that our minds don't allow mothers to feel labor pains when they recall delivering their babies. In like manner, you will remember, but not *feel* again the fear and pain of your surgery or even the discomfort and fatigue of cancer treatments with their side effects. Hurrah for modern medication!

Hospital Admission: One of the first things to happen after you have been admitted to a hospital for surgery and before you are sedated is that someone will bring you an Informed Consent form. By obtaining one before your surgery date, you will be able to present it in completed form immediately upon your arrival. This form will include the name of the doctor and the surgical procedure to be administered. It will state that you have been advised about the risks of surgery and possible blood transfusions. Further, it will mention that any tissue or parts removed by the surgeon will be thoroughly examined.

Informed Consent: Do not be intimidated by this form. It is only a safeguard for the hospital personnel, assuring them and you that you understand what you have read and approve its contents. Be certain that you do understand what it says before signing it. If any part of it is unclear, you should request further information. The form reaffirms that you, the patient, are fully aware of the procedure itself and its risks and have given your voluntary consent to its completion. It basically is a release that protects the doctors and the hospital staff if something unforeseen happens during the procedure.

Prep Instructions: Preparation for breast surgery usually includes having nothing to eat or drink after the midnight before your scheduled surgery. If you have been told that your regular morning pills may be taken, sip as little water as possible. You will be instructed to wear cotton underpants or no underwear at all. This is because synthetic materials might react adversely to some of the electrical instruments being used during surgery. You must leave your eyeglasses or contacts, dentures, and all jewelry at home or with the person who drives you to the hospital. Your armpit may be shaved if any of your lymph nodes are to be removed.

Prep Monitoring: From pre-surgery to your dismissal you will be carefully monitored. Nurses will measure your blood pressure with a cuff around your arm and your blood oxygen with a clip on your finger. They also will keep an eye on your anesthesia in addition to an electrocardiograph which records your heart rate. One soothing procedure may be an electrically warmed blanket that makes you feel pampered. It should help alleviate your normal anxiety along with making you more comfortable in the chill of the hospital room.

Prep Questions: Once you are wearing your hospital gown, you will begin meeting many busy people who will ask you numerous questions. Your anesthesiologist will come to meet you, take your medical history, and reassure you. Many similar questions must be asked repeatedly by various staff members in order to protect you. Be aware of their needs and be patient as well as completely frank. No one will be judging your answers regarding pertinent information. Questions may include whether you:

+have any allergies
+smoke or chew tobacco
+are a heavy drinker of alcohol
+use any drugs or other substances
+have problems with circulation, respiration, or any vital organs

If you have questions to ask, you will be answered in a manner that you can understand. Your surgeon will stop by briefly to chat and to share a bedside conversation that inspires confidence in you that all is well. Nurses will ask if you want to visit the toilet before your IV is inserted. The sensible answer is "Yes," even though later they will accompany you to the bathroom with your attached IV pole in case you change your mind.

Write "Yes": While you are being prepared for surgery, you will be asked many times, "Which breast is having surgery today?" It may seem extreme, but the double-checking should be most comforting to you since you soon will be anesthetized. You also will possibly see one member of your team approaching your side with a magic marker. Strange as it may seem, she will write "Yes" above the breast needing surgery. This idea became standard practice after one horrified doctor inadvertently removed the wrong foot from one of his patients. Today that tragedy can be avoided due to this well-advised procedure.

Vitamin E and Aspirin: Someone must have already told you not to take vitamin E, aspirin, or any blood thinner before surgery. If no one has suggested this advice to you, consider it emphasized now.

OPERATION BEGINS

You will recall being wheeled into the operating room even though you may already have begun to feel the effects of the IV medication. You may remember very little after moving onto the surgery table, for the drugs will put you to sleep almost instantly. You will be unconscious throughout the surgery and will feel no pain.

OPERATION COMPLETED

When you awaken in your recovery bed following the operation, expect to be rather sleepy for a short time. After being wheeled from the recovery area to your scheduled room, you may be given some fruit juice. Soon the nurses will allow you trips to the bathroom. Hospital policy may require an attendant to accompany you with your IV whenever you walk. You may think you are strong enough to walk alone, but you probably are not. Even when you are discharged, a member of the staff will push your wheelchair to your automobile. Sit back and enjoy being spoiled a bit.

POST OPERATION

Anesthesia: Don't think that you are catching a cold after surgery. It's far more likely that the anesthesia left you with frequent sneezes, a runny nose, or a slightly sore throat. These sedative effects can mirror the onset of a cold in your sinus cavities.

Chills: Due to the stress of surgery, your body may react adversely with chills and uncontrollable shakes following the operation. Sometimes, unlike chills from cold temperatures, this trembling may be only inside while your exterior may appear to be completely calm. Gradually, these shaky sensations will subside as you rest and give in to needed sleep.

Don'ts: Medications that were used for sedation during your surgery will remain in your body for at least 24 hours. Actually, following any anesthesia you should drink no alcohol, operate no power tools or any machinery, drive no vehicles, and pilot no airplanes. Just realize that your common sense is not functioning too well. Why not go to sleep and try to enjoy the forced rest?

First Days: The first four or five days following surgery may find you in near-total bed rest. Don't spend too many hours abed after that time. You certainly don't need to add pneumonia or atrophy to your weakened body's primary job of returning you to normal activities.

Shunt: Following surgery, you may be temporarily fitted with a fluid drain called a shunt. It is a tube that has a collection container. The surgeon will insert the tube into your side through a small opening in the skin. The container will be on the outside of your body. You will be given instructions regarding the care of both the drain and your body.

Surgery Arm: If your surgery was for breast cancer and involved removing any lymph nodes, never ever allow *anyone* to take your blood pressure or have blood drawn from your affected arm without permission from your oncologist. If you had operations on both breasts, nurses should try to do all blood work using your legs instead of either arm.

Why Further Treatment: Does your surgeon recommend that you will need more treatment once the tumor itself is removed? Your life certainly would be less interrupted if you did nothing more. The reason for additional treatment is that the cancer possibly has managed to intrude other parts of your body. Surgery definitely makes metastasis less likely to occur, but chemotherapy and/or radiation will further reduce possible risks. Your life is a mighty big gamble if you don't avail yourself of all that modern medicine offers. A delayed decision could cause additional and even more aggressive treatment for your recovery chances. Don't hesitate to continue treatment if it is recommended.

Chapter 4

Chemotherapy

EXPLAINING TREATMENT

Your election to accept chemotherapy should make for a joyful acknowledgement of thanks by your family and friends. Since any hidden cancer cells remaining in your breast will begin to grow again between treatments, each ensuing visit will cause them to shrink. Given periodically in a planned form, chemo works dramatically. The first treatment is especially powerful because the timing and the individually prescribed drugs reduce the malignant cells approximately by half. Each session thereafter tends to do the same. At the time of your final treatment, they can no longer duplicate themselves because they no longer exist!

PREPARATION

Chemo Details: Chemo treatments are relatively painless in their delivery, but you should anticipate spending a couple or three hours at the center if you are an outpatient. Bring something to read or plan to doze. A jacket or a sweater can be a welcomed comfort. Depending on their medication, some cancer patients require hospitalization during their treatment. Oncology nurses will be caring for you and explaining anything you do not understand. Before each treatment, patients will be weighed and given a complete blood count (CBC). Ask for a copy of the results if you keep personal records of your procedures. Also, before each treatment you may expect an individual appointment with your oncologist. Bring with you any written questions for your doctor and/or a tape recorder if you wish.

Chemo Series: Chemotherapy is usually given in a well-spaced series or cycle of treatments followed by days of blessed rest and healing. The timing and blending of chemicals each person receives will often vary considerably among individuals.

Chemo Treatment: Realize that you may need to return to your clinic or oncology office sometime between treatments for daily shots, perhaps extra IVs, or even blood transfusions if needed. This isn't unusual, so don't be frightened; things are still going along fine with your care. It means only that you need a little special attention for a while. The procedures will not only increase your red and white blood cells and platelets, but will also lessen any fatigue. Hopefully you will be one of the people not needing any of these extra *perks*; but if you do need them, be cooperative.

Port—Ask Doctor: Many chemo patients may consider having a port into which their medications will be received. The port will protect your veins from trauma during frequent sessions of chemotherapy. The most available site for its location will be under the collarbone farthest from the surgical incision.

Port—Description: Some surgeons may order a local anesthesia so that the port can be inserted while you are awake. Other doctors may prefer to put you to sleep. Afterwards the skin will hurt a bit for a couple of days, but over-the-counter pain medications should be treatment enough. Your first chemo session could occur immediately after the port is in place. If you were unconscious during its placement, this might be good timing because you will still be groggy and therefore less anxious as you accustom yourself to receiving IVs through the port.

Port—Details: Approximately an inch in diameter, the port will be placed completely inside your body. There will be a small unobtrusive bulge under your skin. The port allows access into a vein just below your collarbone and above your heart. The top or external part of the port accepts medication, while the bottom is attached to a flexible catheter leading into a vein. A certified clinical nurse, using a special needle, will then be able to administer virtually painless injections through your port.

Port—Physical Activity: After insertion of a port, ask your doctor before engaging in sports such as swimming, golfing, or any other physical activity which could possibly cause injury or complications to your treatment.

Port—What to Wear: Port recipients should consider selecting an old comfortable button-up shirt to wear during each chemo treatment. The iodine used as an antiseptic around your port site could stain your good clothing. When your treatments are done, either toss the shirt away or save it for gardening or painting jobs.

MISCELLANEOUS—ANEMIA

Insufficient Oxygen: Red blood cells carry oxygen from the lungs to all parts of your body. Since chemo lowers the number of your red blood cells, the result is that you may get an insufficient amount of oxygen. Called anemia, this condition causes people extreme fatigue. Help is available the moment you speak up. Always report these first signs of energy loss.

Often: Anemia is experienced by over fifty percent of people undergoing chemo. Your doctor will probably arrange for you to have weekly shots to combat this condition. You may still have a few "senior moments" if you are in your retirement years, but you shouldn't blame every memory slip on the cancer treatments! Oh, why not!

Red Spots: Physicians noticing small purple or red spots on a patient's skin may suspect petechiae (puh-tee-kee-eye). These are often the first symptoms of a low platelet count. They are usually discovered during your CBC tests, which are generally given five to seven days after each chemo treatment. Daily shots may be prescribed until the count is elevated to the proper level and the eruptions have disappeared.

Symptoms: Signs of anemia are characterized by feelings of weakness, dizziness, fatigue, chills, irritability and/or shortness of breath. Report any of these symptoms to a nurse even if you aren't scheduled to see your doctor right away.

MISCELLANEOUS — OTHER

Bone Marrow: Chemotherapy drugs affect bone marrow, which in turn lowers your white blood count. This is the main reason that people undergoing cancer treatments are especially prone to infections. It is encouraging to realize that, generally speaking, the drugs you will be given destroy bad cells and disturb the good ones only temporarily.

Combination of Drugs: Your treatments will include a combination of powerful anti-cancer drugs because they have been proven more effective than relying on a single drug. Over a period of months, these treatments are given in cycles with each followed by a recovery period before the start of the next. Both the medications and the amount of time you will need them are prescribed for you individually.

Dermatologist: After a few chemo treatments, sometimes the chemicals work from the inside out, thereby alleviating the need to visit dermatologists during treatments. How about that for a *good* side effect!

Laboratory Blood Work: Avoid excessive bruising after having blood drawn from your veins by refraining from lifting or carrying any heavy object (including your all-purpose purse) for several hours.

Lymphedema-Common Sense: Members of your health team may say that you don't have to worry about lymphedema because you had so few lymph nodes removed during surgery. Take precautions anyway. Sometimes a combination of surgery and radiation will activate swelling. No one knows your body the way you do. Use common sense and be on the alert for any heaviness or aches in your surgery arm. If you suspect any trouble in that arm, ask your doctor to recommend a therapist who can teach you how to do some massages, light rotating *skin wiggles,* and other helpful techniques.

Measuring Lymphedema: Periodic medical measuring of arms and legs is one way for a comparison check against lymphedema, which is a collection of fluid causing swelling.

Preventing Lymphedema: To treat or help prevent lymphedema:

+Never get shots, have blood pressure checked, or have blood drawn on the arm nearer the surgery site if any lymph nodes have been removed.

+Protect that arm from injury, infection, sunburn, and insect bites.

+Lift only light objects (under five pounds) with that arm.

+Carry your shoulder bag or purse with your unaffected arm.

+Use only an electric razor if you shave underarms.

+Don't wear tight jewelry or elastic blouses or jackets.

Treating Lymphedema: If you develop lymphedema, seek help immediately since early treatment is vital to early relief. Treatment often includes exercises and massages with restrictive physical therapy, plus compression elastic sleeves. Also elevating the affected area, avoiding salt, and using diuretic medications are likely to be prescribed to avoid a chronic situation.

Shots—Epoetin Alpha (e.g. Procrit): Procrit is a drug that builds red blood cells to control anemia.

If needed, be glad to take these shots because they are designed specifically to help you become physically stronger. We all want that quality of life as long as possible. Incidentally, Procrit shots really can hurt if injected too swiftly. You may need to request tactfully that any unfamiliar nurse please inject them slowly.

Shots—Filgrastim (e.g. Neupogen): Your oncologist may order daily Neupogen shots or other similar drugs for a few weeks after chemo treatments. These shots may cause your bones to ache for several days thereafter. They are vital in helping you avoid a low white cell count, sometimes called low blood. This condition could cause you to become particularly prone to infection. You are required to show up for the total chemo series even if you're feeling terrible. Besides boosting your immune system, the shots will soon help you feel better and raise your spirits. They are literally and figuratively a shot in the arm!

Shots—Friends: One bonus in all cancer treatments, from shots and IVs to x-rays and waiting rooms, is that you will develop friends whose schedule will be about the same as yours. Most folks are eager to share their mutual side effects and to offer or receive suggestions on how to ease them. These are the people who will truly understand your continuing journey toward recovery.

Shots—Relax: No one enjoys having injections, but try to relax as much as possible. Needles go into skin tissue much more readily when muscles are not tense and tight. One trick to get your mind and eyes off the shots is to concentrate on humming to yourself or wiggling your toes while relaxing your muscles at the same time. You will hardly notice the needle.

Water, the Best Liquid: Drugs tend to crystallize in your kidneys if they aren't flushed out regularly. Of all liquids, water is the best. This is especially important right after chemo treatments. Eight to ten servings a day sounds like a lot, but when your mouth is dry, water goes down fine! Be sure you keep a few bottles of fresh water around the house and in your car. Some people think that you will drink more if you sip through a straw.

Water—Drink Plenty: Both chemotherapy and radiation affect your entire body from tip to toe. They alter skin and inner organs, ridding you of all imperfections as well as some healthy cells. Knowing this surely encourages people to do whatever possible to rebuild any depletion as best they can with plenty of water and nutritious food. An unexpected benefit of chemo is that skin blemishes and pre-cancers seem to disappear from the inner treatments to the outer skin surfaces. Magic!

Water—Urine: Immediately after having chemo treatment, don't be surprised if certain chemical injections cause your urine to be red for a few hours. Some other drugs cause a strong urine odor to last for a long time; however, consuming a lot of water will dilute the oily-looking discolored urine and also reduce much of the vile odor. Incidentally, if your urine is very yellow, your body is telling you to drink more liquids.

Chapter 5

Radiation

PREPARATIONS

Chemo and/or Radiation: Sometimes doctors use radiation before surgery to shrink a tumor. For other patients, it may be given after or even during chemotherapy. All cancer treatments are individualized based especially on the stage and location of the tumor. As a consequence, therapy and various side effects deviate considerably from one patient to another.

CT "CAT" Scan—Iodine Allergy: Iodine-containing materials are sometimes used in these scans. If you are allergic to iodine and are scheduled for this procedure, be certain to report that information to your radiology team.

CT "CAT" Scan—Painless: This scan may or may not take a long time, depending upon the need for the procedure. It is not painful, except for the mental anguish of having to lie perfectly still for an undetermined length of time. Trust that all is going as it should when some of the mechanical equipment occasionally makes weird noises and seems to have developed periodic hiccups.

Dosage: With many types of cancer, radiation is generally given five days a week for six or seven weeks. Of course this cyclical dosage is individually prescribed. When possible, many small daily amounts of radiation are given rather than a few large doses, thereby protecting more normal tissue in the tumor area. Fortunately, weekend rest periods allow the patient as well as normal cells to begin recovering.

Immobilization Device: Radiation therapists are more than careful; they are obsessive! Since these rays may be delivered to the same area for only one series, you will begin with planning periods called simulations. An immobilization device like a plastic molded pillow will be formed to help you remain still and in exactly the same specified place during each treatment. You will want to be sure to wear slacks and heavy socks for these simulations, as it is quite cold on those flat beds. Neither these preliminary preparations nor any of the radiation procedures themselves is the least bit painful.

PREPARATIONS — MARKINGS

Ink: One must not rub the marks or try to remove them when showering, for the therapists need them as guides. Eventually the inked lines will fade and need to be re-marked a number of times until all your treatments are finished. Only then are you able to allow them to disappear naturally as time passes on. Sorry, but you shouldn't expect to see any beautiful butterflies or personal slogans at all from any of these markings or tattoos.

Stains: Before washing ink-stained clothing, applying hair spray seems to help remove the discoloration.

Tattoo: The perimeters of your cancer area will be indicated with magic markers and/or dye injections like tiny tattooed dots to ensure a perfect alignment for the application of the rays. The therapists will put special blocks between the machine and certain parts of your body to protect normal tissues and organs. It is gratifying to know that these blocks and markings are the precise areas stipulated by your radiologist. That is the primary concern of these professionals who are also perfectionists.

Tattoo Substitutes: Some radiologists haven't been using tattoos for all patients. Instead, between sessions they mark their measured areas more extensively with various colored inks and cover the marks with tape. This protects the markings from fading as you take your daily showers.

PREPARATIONS — OTHER

Monitor: Before the radiation therapists actually begin the five to ten minute treatments, they will leave the room. As they monitor the machine, they can both see and hear you the entire time. The equipment can be stopped at any point, so if you feel uncomfortable, ill, or anticipate a cough or a sneeze, tell them at once.

Words You'll Hear: During radiation treatments, you'll become accustomed to hearing certain words frequently. These statements and their reasons are explained below:

> "Don't help as we move you into position." The therapists will pull the sheet underneath you and move you infinitesimally to align you with their measurements for the machine.
> "Try to stay very still now." You must remain as immobile as you can during the treatment so radiation reaches exactly where it is needed and to the same area with each treatment.
> "Okay, here we go." Prepare to lie absolutely still until the therapists return to your side.
> "Sit on the side of the table a moment before getting down." Often you'll feel momentary dizziness when you first sit up.

"Your appointment is for ?:00 tomorrow."
Some people need to be seen twice a day
with six hours in between treatments.
Appointment times frequently vary from
day to day.

X—Rays: You will have frequent pictures taken
of your treatment areas. These x-rays will allow
your physician to evaluate your progress through
comparisons with earlier pictures. This duplication
process will assure the therapists that they are
following the precisely marked guidelines.

MISCELLANEOUS

Deodorants: Expect the radiologist to advise you
throughout your treatments to forgo any underarm
deodorants or the new powdered sunscreens.

Earaches: Some people who receive treatments
experience hardening of ear wax which may produce
earaches. Unless you have radiation to the neck or
head, wax buildup is only an indirect cause of the
trouble. More likely the fatigue brought on by your
treatments results in less stamina. With this decrease
in energy, you'll naturally become less attentive to
your normal bodily care.

Esophagus: If radiation treatments must touch
your esophagus, you will undoubtedly develop a sore
throat. You must report it and then relief will be
forthcoming.

Skin Burns: If you experience burns, be sure to check with your doctor before buying any ointment to ensure that the alcohol content is minimal. The gels are thick and tend to adhere to your clothing as well as to your skin. The lotions are smooth moisturizers that can be used after treatments and at bedtime. Neither the gels nor the moisturizers are allowed to be used four hours prior to your radiation treatments.

Skin Discoloration: You should expect some darkening and possibly delayed burning or blistering of the skin areas following radiation. Never use cold packs against these affected areas.

Skin Itch: During radiation, your skin will become red or may darken as the pigmentation temporarily changes. If you need relief, ask your therapist to suggest something that will ease pains and itching skin.

Skin Lotions: You must avoid the sun and use no sunscreen until radiation therapy is completed. If your treated areas begin to itch, a light coating of cornstarch may help. Do not apply any creams or lotions without the approval of the health team, and then only during the specified hours before daily treatments. Many lotions can leave a coating that might interfere with the rays. Ask questions if you have any doubts at all.

Skin Pain: Although radiation burns your skin in a way which is similar to sunburn, receiving the beams is totally painless. The use of aloe gels and lotions help immensely to soothe these areas. Carefully read labels on ointments in order to select those that contain the least alcohol content.

Skin Tingles: At the beginning of radiation there is very little discoloration, but with further treatments your skin will darken. Occasionally it may burn, but ointments will be offered by your health team. Healing will begin soon after the treatments end. What sometimes may last for many months thereafter are uncomfortable tingles under the skin that feel like creepy crawlers.

Tingling Digits: If you are a patient who suffers from neuropathy, a malfunction of the nerves often causing tingling and/or numbness of your fingers and toes, the addition of vitamin B6 in your diet could help. At the very least, it is worth mentioning to your health caregiver.

Vitamins: After radiation ends, it is important to supplement your diet with lots of calcium and water. Vitamins also are important in helping you regain your previous state of everyday good health.

SUPPLEMENTAL

Immune Disorders: It is not uncommon for autoimmune disorders such as fibromyalgia, lupus, or arthritis to flare up during radiation treatments. Notify oncologists and any doctors treating these other ailments. The right hand must know what the left hand is doing.

Palliative Care: Curing cancer is not always possible, so radiation therapy is frequently used to shrink tumors and reduce pressure, pain, and other symptoms. When radiation is used for such palliative care, cancer patients usually have a longer and better quality of life.

Survivor: Remember that radiation and your chemo drugs are doing battle for you, taking away the power of the enemy cancer. Vow to be a survivor!

UPDATE — BRACHYTHERAPY

Brachytherapy Implants: Never abandon hope! New treatments are being found every day. One of the latest new hopes for breast tumor patients is a form of brachytherapy. This procedure, a relatively new word to most people outside the medical community, delivers radiation into the body by means of an implantation in the form of needles or seeds. The implants are left for a specified amount of time, with some being removed in a few days while others may remain permanently.

Hope: Brachytherapy implantation has already been used successfully for some head and neck cancers. By increasing dosage directly into the tumor, this therapy can be given either before or after the more familiar external beam method. Sometimes doctors are using this treatment even for cervix, uterine, and prostate treatments.

Mammosite: The future may find more types of cancer patients, including those with breast cancer, who may benefit from brachytherapy as an alternative treatment. The National Cancer Institute (NCI) originated a plan to monitor the feasibility of using a MammoSite device. Its function was to place a radioactive seed inside the breast which may allow external radiation time to be reduced or eliminated altogether. *Hope springs eternally!*

WELFARE OF OTHERS

Having external radiation beams cannot make anyone radioactive.

Chapter 6

Side Effects

A LIST OF POSSIBLE SIDE EFFECTS

Aches

Appetite loss

Backaches

Bleeding

Breathing problems

Burns

Clothing that fits

Dental problems

Diarrhea

Dizziness

Edema/Fluid retention

Eye problems

Anemia

Arm awareness

Balance

Breast changes

Bruising

Chills

Constipation

Depression

Discoloration

Ear discomfort

Energy loss

Fever

Fatigue

Fluid retention/Swelling

Headaches

Hot Flashes

Infections

Irritability

Lactose intolerance

Mental instability

Muscular aches

Nausea/Stomach/
    Vomiting

Numbness

Phlegm increases

Rash

Stomach problems

Swallowing/Throat
    problems

Taste bud changes

Urine discoloration

Vision changes

Weakness

Finger and Toe
    irregularities

Hair loss

Hormonal changes

Immune disorders

Insomnia

Itch

Memory loss

Mouth problems

Nail changes

Nose/Odor sensitivity

Pain

Pores enlarged

Skin difficulties

Stress

Swelling

Throat discomfort

Vaginal dryness

Vomiting

Weight changes

Of course this looks like a terrifying list. It is always very important to stress that, while you may never have many of these side effects, some will occur just occasionally. Those that you do experience will be lessened when you follow your doctors' prescribed medications and their suggestions to modify them.

APPETITE

Dietician: Having no appetite is one of the most annoying side effects you are likely to face. If you need suggestions or have any dietary questions, visit any American Cancer Society (ACS) office and make an appointment with their clinical outpatient dietitian. You'll find them extremely knowledgeable, amiable, and helpful.

Improvement: About ten days after each chemo, your appetite will improve until the next treatment. Try to use this period of grace to increase your amount of food intake gradually. During your recovery, it will probably take less time for your body to adjust to your former routine.

Metallic Taste: One of the chief reasons that many patients have poor appetites is due to a metallic taste. Sucking any hard candy helps some people. Using the Altoids brand citrus and tangerine flavors may be preferred since they don't have the chalky sensation of many other mints. Also, the citric acid leaves a slightly sour taste which seems to take away the disagreeable problem for longer periods of time.

Mouth: Oddly, what tastes good after one treatment may be replaced by a quite different taste after the next session. Of course you must be very much aware that your body also is changing and that may account for some of your new food choices.

BATHROOM

Constipation: There is danger in straining too much with constipation. One man strained too long one morning and found himself on the tile floor with a goose egg bump on his forehead. Strokes can also be caused by over-straining. The number of early morning sirens may attest to that fact.

Diarrhea: If diarrhea is your problem of the moment, check with your physician to see what remedy may be recommended.

Flush Often: Except for warm showers, bathroom trips are unpleasant for sensitive noses. Just learn to flush often, even before you are ready to stand up!

Reading Material: Keep reading material within reach in your home's "rest room" in case it becomes your "waiting room" during any bouts with diarrhea or constipation.

Stomach Cramps: Warning: if you develop stomach cramps after eating, go without hesitation directly to the bathroom to avoid accidents. Some surprises are no fun!

CHILLS

Sometimes sudden chills may occur with cancer treatment, so have a sweater handy whenever you leave your home. If you do suddenly get chills with a fever, however, consult your doctors pronto. They need to know about anything that is irregular or worrisome to you. After determining whether or not the symptoms are related to your treatment, they will be able to prescribe a remedy. When your problems are not an expected side effect, the doctors will treat you accordingly.

FATIGUE

Depression: If you experience extreme fatigue and/or depression due to any treatment, your oncologist must be told. The suggested help may include taking several naps per day in addition to your moderate exercise. You may also be told to eat a snack every few hours rather than only at set mealtimes. Many side effects can be lessened.

Energy: Your energy levels will fluctuate as your white blood count rises and falls. Being aware of this possibility makes you realize that it is a natural side effect of treatments. If your WBC is too low, you will feel washed out. Make your health team aware of your ebbing energy so that they may help you feel better right away.

Naps: When fatigue hits, give in to it and take a nap, which should revive you. Except for your medical appointments, everything else can wait!

Tears: Occasional tears are normal; just don't allow yourself to drown in them.

HAIR

Nightcap: When your hair is gone, you will probably want a nightcap - not an alcoholic nightcap, but some soft apparel to keep your head warm. It will feel good to wear around the house as well as during sleep. You will awaken without a hangover, guaranteed!

Recovery: The growth of your new hair will be slow but more exciting than any roller coaster ride; it is the first truly visible sign that you are regaining your health. Many women in recovery find that some straight hair grows back curly, but it usually returns to its normal straight pattern as soon as it is cut. If you have naturally curly hair, will it come back straight? It may even change color. You can't be sure until it begins to return.

Soft: Your new growth of hair may be baby soft and, after being with none at all for such a long time, it will feel wonderful to your touch. It may remain quite short for many months, but you'll be fascinated by the restoration process.

HAIR & SKIN

First the hair and skin are affected when subjected to chemotherapy and radiation, but the good news is that subsequently they are renewed more quickly than other parts of the body.

INFECTIONS

Avoid: Infections can be dangerous for cancer patients. Your treatments are known to lower your white blood count which weakens and destroys your body's natural defenses against outside invasions. It may be wise to wash your hands and brush your teeth more often than usual. Infections can rapidly become serious if not arrested immediately. The temptation to pay no heed to them is especially strong over weekends. Never ignore even slight infections without both treating and reporting them. If fever develops, get emergency help.

Crowds: After being forced indoors for long periods of time, many folks may become stir crazy. Of course, there is some legitimate fear of possible infections or flu when you join crowds. Taking a car ride around town or to the beach, mountains, or woods is a safer option. Even short outings allow you to feel part of everyday life again.

Toothbrush Care & Replacement: Just as you are to wash your hands often to avoid mouth infections, also take care either to boil your toothbrush or to put it into the dishwasher weekly. During this time, the importance of tossing out old toothbrushes more frequently is as significant as it is when recovering from head colds. Perhaps at bedtime, the night after each chemo treatment, would be an easy way to remember to replace your toothbrush for the sake of safety.

INSOMNIA

If you are troubled with insomnia, consider preparing for bed soon after your evening meal. In that way, when you begin feeling sleepy, you can lie down immediately. Beware of late-night TV movies. They may stimulate your interest too much for you to want to go back to sleep. However, if you awaken in the middle of the night, you may enjoy trying lighter fare, such as the animal programs which are on 24/7. The segments are short enough to finish in half an hour. Flip the OFF button during commercials before the next episode can tempt you. Probably bed will feel good enough by then to lull you back into dreamland.

KNOWLEDGE

Reading the cancer material offered by oncologists can be frightening until you understand that all the side effects mentioned do not mean that you will experience each of them. Hospitals need to make full disclosure of possible side effects in order to insulate themselves from potential non-disclosure liability. Granted, much of what you will read or be told will be scary, but realize that whatever side effects each individual may develop will vary in intensity.

NAILS

Changes: One side effect that some people experience is actually good. Finger nails sometimes grow longer and stronger than before treatment. The down side is that once treatment ends, the nails begin to soften and are prone to split or peel for several months into recovery. What do you suppose that is all about anyway? An oddity worthy of show and tell, that's what!

Discoloration: Another strange side effect which folks occasionally find is having their finger and toe nails grow darker than they did before chemo. After treatments end, the nails recover, chameleon-like; from the roots to the tips, the discoloration slowly grows out and normal tissue returns. While the process is pleasant, watching the unnatural colors diminish assures you that the toxins are finally being expelled.

REPORT

Duty: Due to the many side effects during cancer care, oncologists and their assistants thoroughly and regularly monitor each patient. Still, it is up to you to report any conditions that concern you. It is very normal to need frequent assurance that all is proceeding properly.

Weekend: If a disturbing question or problem occurs to you over a holiday or weekend, as they often seem to do, your oncologist may be unavailable for calls. In that case look online, contact a pharmacist, find a clinic, or go to an emergency room for comforting answers. Checking with someone for the sake of your own health will also ease your peace of mind.

SKIN

Discoloration: Everyone reacts differently to treatments, yet many side effects are shared by all. Surprisingly, as the body changes with each treatment, so do some of the side effects. Skin coloring is often one of the most obvious changes as it develops more shades. Sometimes, if your skin is light and becomes too dark, it may seem like a curse. Other times, when it makes you less pale, you appear quite healthy and then the changes become a welcomed blessing.

Pores: Some chemo treatments cause large pores to appear on your face; other treatments do the exact opposite and are great for they make your skin look and feel as smooth as a newborn baby's. That is a side effect you hope will remain forever.

STRESS

Stress is your enemy, especially when your body is already being attacked. Try to forestall potentially troublesome situations and actively avoid confronting as many problems as possible. Even small problems loom large when you aren't feeling tiptop.

TENDENCY

Although you may never suffer some of the bad side effects mentioned in brochures or elsewhere, individuals experience certain effects that tend to recur after each treatment. You'll learn to identify and cope with your own.

TRIGGER

Cancer treatment can trigger your arthritis or any other physical weakness. After all, the medication flows throughout your entire body. Mention this or any other unexpected problems to your health team.

UNUSUAL OR SEVERE SIDE EFFECTS

All medications need to be carefully monitored by you and your physician. If either you or your caregiver notice any unusual ill effects, it is imperative that you notify your oncologist at once. Prescription amounts vary with individuals. Often any dosage can be readjusted to meet a particular need. Any extreme sign of side effects as mentioned previously should definitely be reported, but special attention must be given immediately if any of the following symptoms occur during your treatment:

Disorientation
Eyes or skin yellowing
Hallucinations
Mental instability

Mood changes

Nightmares

The chances of anyone developing any of these severe side effects during your treatment are extremely unlikely; if, however, they do occur be sure to contact your doctor promptly so counteraction may be taken at once.

Chapter 7

Recovery

TREATMENT — TAMOXIFEN

Hormonal Therapy: Tamoxifen, a frequently prescribed hormone treatment, is used to prevent the recurrence of breast cancers since many of them grow in response to estrogen. It blocks the use of estrogen in any cancerous cells that may remain in the breast. It is a daily pill frequently prescribed for the five years following chemotherapy and radiation treatment, but it does not stop the body's production of estrogen. Some symptoms it may cause include hot flashes, a painful vaginal discharge, irritation, or nausea; nevertheless, serious side effects are rare. You should feel optimistic since many people have no Tamoxifen side effects whatsoever.

Menses: For women who are still having menstrual periods and are sexually active, their form of birth control should be condoms or diaphragms rather than birth control pills. The effects of Tamoxifen may alter the development of a fetus. In addition, these women could have irregular periods and may become pregnant more easily when taking Tamoxifen. Doctors will regularly want to see any patient whose uterus is still intact.

New Generic Inhibitors: Some newly released inhibitors, Letrozole (e.g. Femara) and Anastrozole (e.g. Arimidex), may offer hope in reducing the possible ill effects of prolonged use of Tamoxifen. The standard treatment has been for some post menopausal women to take Tamoxifen daily for as long as five years. Many doctors are now recommending that it be used for just two to three years followed by taking other medications during the final period of hormonal treatment. Further advanced inhibitors will no doubt be offered to the public as they are developed and approved.

TREATMENT — TAMOXIFEN :

Scientists: There are some scientists who now think that Tamoxifen may increase the odds of the development of both uterine and breast cancers. Still, this pill is prescribed in hopes of a lasting warranty against a return of any cancer. Some physicians may prescribe similar drugs instead of Tamoxifen.

MISCELLANEOUS

Appointments: The time to make appointments for checkups with all your regular physicians will be soon after your final treatment. These follow-ups usually include examination of chest, neck, underarm areas, both breasts, and measuring of the surgery arm, as well as periodic mammograms of one or both breasts. (Special techniques can be used for women with breast implants.) Another recommended follow-up after radiation is related to any needed dental work. Problems are prone to develop after some of your therapy, especially if you have been allowed to have only urgent dental work throughout your treatment.

Clothing: If your weight changes dramatically, you may need to buy a whole new wardrobe and give your old clothing to a thrift shop. Donations may be worth at least five or ten dollars each, so you might want a receipt which may allow you to have a deduction at tax time.

Energy: During your early recovery from cancer, tell your friends in advance that your energy may suddenly fade. This will help them understand and not be offended when you need to cut short their visits. Even during recovery, visits of more than 30 minutes can be very tiring.

Exercise: At some point after removal of your lymph nodes, you may suffer from muscular tightness or pains in your arms or shoulders that shout, "Help needed here!" Inform your doctor in order that you may soon be working out with trained physical therapists. They will be able to show you how to protect yourself from possible injuries caused by inexperience. The more moderate exercise you do, the better you will feel. It's not all fun and games even if they do have neat machines, huge exercise balls, stretch bands, and massage rooms. Just work hard with the therapist and also at home in order to recover amazingly fast.

Fatigue: During your recovery phase, light exercise, adequate food and water, and frequent naps are important. Always pay close attention to your body. It is very tempting to overdo when unaccustomed energy levels are high again, however sometimes fatigue can return rapidly and cause your body to demand that you pace your activities.

Fear of Mental Shutdown: Once a woman's appetite has returned and he has begun eating regularly, a sudden lack of desire for food may be a sign of fading hope. During her recovery period, a total disinterest in eating indicates one of the most significant signs of a patient's mental decline. It may be an unconscious desire to give up rather than to continue treatment. Family or caregivers should consider seeking a psychologist who treats depression and may be able to help her revive her natural inclination to survive this low phase.

Freezer: Remember to stock your freezer with small and simple meals that may appeal to you at odd moments as your health improves and your taste buds begin returning to normal.

Hair — Compassion: As your own hair grows back and body scars fade, you will have developed more compassion and understanding for new patients.

Hair — Fun: If you lose your hair, as many people do, you will find it fascinating and fun to notice the varying patterns of growth as it returns. It's amazing how your hair knows just which way to run so that your head will be completely covered. It will feel so good to you when it returns that you can hardly keep your fingers away from it!

Lotions: As a recovering patient, it will be suggested that you continue applying aloe lotions daily for the remainder of your life. It will help keep radiated skin soft and stretchy. Used after warm showers, it also will keep your skin from becoming dry, flaky and scaly, just as it did during your radiation therapy. Smoother skin is definitely healthier and more comfortable.

Mouth: Some of the last things to disappear during recovery are bad aftertastes and recurring dry mouths. The good news is that both of these annoyances improve with each passing day.

Patience: Some milder effects of cancer treatment extend into many months after the end of regulated treatments. Expecting that will enable you to notice and enjoy the gradual disappearance of each adverse effect. Yea!

Sense of Fear: Throughout the recovery phase, you will realize there is an underlying fear of a recurrence, along with an additional concern regarding the ability of friends and family to be supportive once again. *If* there is a recurrence, when you had hoped all treatments were finished, you will dread further treatment and especially the thought of still more cancer cells to conquer.

Sense of Loss: As wonderful as finishing treatment makes you feel, you will also notice a sense of loss of the routine scheduling to which you have become accustomed. Along with the end of treatment comes the end of relationships you have developed with many caring doctors, nurses, and fellow patients who have become your friends.

Toenails: If your toenails darkened during chemotherapy, as your recovery continues you may find it fun to follow their gradual return to normalcy. Just glance down and check the color of the nails as you take your daily shower. Once all of the toxins work their way out of your system, you'll be out of the recovery stage and can term yourself a true cancer survivor!

Tolerance: Be prepared for most side effects to lessen but not completely disappear possibly even for years after treatments have ceased. Recovery is so much easier than the effects withstood in your recent past that you can tolerate the present nuisances a bit longer.

True Recovery: Unfortunately, true recovery is not over for many months after the end of treatments. This phase may include follow-up visits to your physicians every three months, plus having a mammogram every six months in addition to occasional x-rays and blood tests. Later, you probably will graduate to six-month checkups and then yearly ones. Although your life has changed forever, the realization that the recovery period is just another cycle of your life may make it less fearful. It can become another important awareness of all human mortality. As the little man, Alfred E. Neumann, says in *MAD Magazine*, "What, me worry?"

Wonder: The battle against cancer is never ending. You will always wonder if all that you have endured means that you have really won. Is this war the complete victory you promised yourself? (Indeed, will any war ever be the end of all wars?) Is the cancer just lurking in some hidden spot, waiting to ambush you after your protective treatments and support systems are gone? In recovery you feel relatively safe again, but the checkups remind you that you must be constantly on guard.

SIDE EFFECTS

Beginning after treatments: Some side effects may begin a number of months after all treatments are completed. Your breast may begin to feel quite firm or a bit swollen. Regular exercise each day plus massaging vitamin E cream into your affected skin is highly recommended to forestall complications. There also is a chance that your skin and the muscles around your treatment and scar areas may begin to tighten, causing your shoulder to ache. Physical therapy, including a series of stretch exercises and massages, may be suggested when you report these problems to your doctor. In order to receive physical therapy, you will need a doctor's prescription.

Continuing too long: Sad to say, but some minor side effects may continue for many years. Usually these are just annoyances such as a lack of feeling in your surgery areas, memory loss, dry mouth, or discoloration of your skin in radiation-treated locations. They are all possible results of your surgery, chemo and/or radiation. As time goes by, these nuisances should gradually diminish, but it may seem frighteningly long to you unless you are pre-warned to expect them to linger.

Chapter 8

Recurrence

ANXIETY

After treatments end, you will be anxious about the possible recurrence of cancer. This is perfectly normal. Of course you should be alert to any unusual signs and report them to your doctor without hesitation. As you regain strength and endurance along with your normal energy level, you should gradually recover from the rigors of your treatments.

FEARS

Treatments are such an emotional drain on both patients and caregivers that a reappearance of any feared signs may become overly stressful for everyone. Patients worry that family and friends will be so worn out from your initial bout that they may be much less supportive of any future recurrence of this disease.

RISK

No one yet has been able to figure out why some folks who seem at high risk for the return of cancer remain free of it, while others who seem to be at lower risk may be fated to suffer more assaults. Apparently it follows that the fewer lymph nodes involved, the lower the chance is of reappearance. The highest likelihood for recurrence is in women who had ten or more malignant nodes removed; however, the odds shrink depending upon the original size of the tumor. They decrease even further if none of the bean-like nodes breaks through their pods and spreads.

TIMING

A recurrence, if any, might appear within two or three years after treatment; but some breast cancers may return many years later if undetected cancer cells begin to multiply after periods of dormancy. Individuals with recurring cancer may have one or a combination of various types of treatment.

UNUSUAL SIDE EFFECTS — POST TREATMENT

Once your treatments are completed, be aware that your risk of any recurrence is unpredictable.

Check with your oncologist if you develop any *excessive* symptoms of those mentioned previously, or any of the ones listed below. By now many of these signs seem somewhat normal, but if they are beyond routine you should seek advice.

+Aches and Pains/Appetite loss
+Breathing problems
+Coughing or hoarseness
+Depression
+Digestive problems
+Disorientation
+Dizziness
+Falling
+Fatigue
+Headaches
+Lumps
+Menstrual changes
+Mental instability
+Vision changes
+Weight variations

Of course these could be just a sign of some temporary problem, but it would be wise to allow an oncologist to make that determination. Just as a safeguard, your physician may order an MRI or other test to check any distressing condition.

Chapter 9

Tips

ARM WARNINGS

Breast cancer patients who have had lymph nodes removed must protect the surgery arm forever. Avoid using that arm to lift items which weigh more than five pounds. Be careful of heavy purses, infants, suitcases, grocery bags, et cetera. Wear long sleeves against extreme cold or intense sunshine. Use insect repellents. Promptly put salves and lotions on injuries, and never allow anyone to use that extra-sensitive arm for taking your blood pressure, injecting shots, or drawing blood.

BACK RUBS

Aloe: When bones ache miserably, back rubs with aloe lotion are most welcome. If they don't volunteer, ask your spouse or a close friend for one.

Back rubs that are lovingly given make sickness itself much easier to tolerate.

Human Touch: There can be great tenderness in the human touch. If your body aches, a gentle back rub feels great when someone who really cares for you does the rubbing. The loving touch seems to flow through their fingertips.

BALANCE

Some treatments make people feel temporarily off balance. Be careful bending over, turning corners when walking from room to room, or rising from a chair too fast, any one of which could cause you suddenly to feel light-headed.

BRASSIERES

Especially right after breast surgery, most women will find that wearing a brassiere to bed makes for easier sleeping. Sports bras are particularly supportive. Following lymph node removal, keeping your surgery arm on a pillow should make you more comfortable. It will also help if you have a shunt or fluid draining tube then and for a time thereafter as your body reclaims its own draining process.

"BYTES GANG "

Most of us are fully qualified for membership in the Bytes Gang* because of frequent insect bites,

*Breaks Your Tender Endangered Skin Gang

thistles and thorns, cuts and burns, scrapes and punctures. We do need to be particularly careful all during treatment and recovery until our immune systems are fully on guard again.

CALL BY NAME

In cancer groups only first names really matter to patients, caregivers, and staff; but using them can make the difference between bonding and just being together for a while. Even if you need to ask a person's name more than once, you will have shown that you really want to remember it. How flattering!

CHILLS

Cancer treatments tend to make people either too hot, or even more often, too cold. Be prepared when you leave your home by carrying a sweater. Socks can also be comforting. Even wigs and turbans can give needed protection against winds and chills.

COMPUTER E-MAIL

Having use of a computer is a big plus for cancer patients. It is much easier to E-mail monthly updates and thank-you notes to family and friends than writing longhand or making phone calls to many people. Thanks to E-mail, one old-fashioned round robin letter can fly through space to many people.

COPING

Positive Attitude: The best way to help your children's future has always been in making sure that your own marriage is good. In like manner, the best way to show other patients that they too can cope with their treatments is by setting a good example in keeping your attitude positive.

Ten Keys:
1. Maintain a positive attitude.
2. Eat even when you don't want *any* food.
3. Practice patience.
4. Do exactly what your doctor recommends, but realize that your body is primarily your own responsibility.
5. Look for small pleasures.
6. Actively participate in helping other people through their rough days.
7. Do something "normal" every day.
8. Know that bad moments will pass.
9. Move around as much as possible; exercising even in simple ways will help you feel better and more in control of yourself.
10. Remember that cancer cells can't stand the treatments, but *you* can!

CROWDS

Keeping out of large crowds is prudent during treatment. Be discriminating, particularly during flu season, in regard to the people with whom you come in contact.

DECISIONS

Alternative Medicines: Some friends will suggest alternative medicines despite the fact that you already have chosen treatment which is comfortable for you. Understand that they care about you enough to suggest procedures which *they* feel are superior to those you have already chosen. Don't be offended by them; feel cherished instead.

Postponement: Life isn't easy. Many of our choices are painful, but prolonging the need to make a decision can cause an even more painful future. Postponing health issues too long is a bad decision in itself.

Relatives: Because it is sometimes hard to concentrate or make important decisions alone, it could be helpful to choose a relative or friend with whom to discuss your options. Verbalizing ideas can help crystallize your thoughts.

DEPRESSION

There will be some surprising times when your spirits drop and your eyes leak for no good reason. A nice cry can keep you from having a sore throat caused by trying to hold back weeping. However, if you are feeling especially blue or discouraged, tell your doctors or nurses. Many medications can cause a feeling of depression. If needed, your medical team can even arrange for you to see a professional to help you cope with your temporary problem. Depression is not a weakness but your body's cry for help. There is no shame in talking with a trained and objective listener.

DIAPERS

It pays to be prepared. Plastic diaper-like slip-on underpants belong in every bathroom for use in case of sudden unexpected side effects. If you never need to use them, count your blessings. You're way ahead of the game.

ENERGY

Bad days: During your "bad" days, reading in bed will either help keep your mind occupied and away from your aches and pains or put you to sleep. Either one will bring an appreciated respite.

Best days: Healing comes with much rest. Remember this on your "best" days and don't overdo. On your "bad" days you will need no reminders!

Conserve: Fatigue is the main side effect most breast cancer patients seem to suffer from their radiation treatments. One of the easiest ways to overcome fatigue, other than napping of course, is to walk extra slowly most of the time until recovery is complete. This means especially to conserve your energy when you are feeling your best. Protecting your fragility can lessen the chances of sudden exhaustion. Consider using a cane for a while even if it makes you look and feel like an invalid; besides, people are less likely to bump into you and cause you to lose your balance.

Handicap parking: If you become weak enough to need a walker or a wheelchair, you may want to pick up a handicap parking form from your motor vehicle department. This form must be signed by your doctor and returned to that department in order to obtain a Handicap Parking Placard.

Handicap vs. non-handicap: Caregivers and friends can help enlighten the public to the fact that cancer patients may need the use of designated handicap parking places for their treatments or other necessary sojourns. People sometimes don't look ill but simply have unseen problems or simply a limited supply of energy. They can become extremely upset when thoughtless citizens deprive them of those special spaces.

Limited: Expect fatigue after the expenditure of your limited energy. Even a fifteen minute rest will do wonders. Simply practice pacing your activities and you'll be fine.

Low platelet count: If your platelet count drops, avoid physical tasks. A vacation from housework or taxing exertion of any kind can be a thing to enjoy, giving you more real time simply to relax and do as little as possible.

Naps: Napping an hour or two in a recliner with the television on is okay. You are still sleeping.

Rest: Even when you feel extra good during cancer treatments, take time to rest enough so you don't use all your energy too quickly.

Strength: Do as much as you are able to do when you feel well, but remember that you aren't up to your full strength, so try to regulate the way you spend your energy.

EXERCISE

Frequently: During some breast surgery, lymph nodes may be removed from your armpits. Start the suggested exercises when your oncologist orders them. They will entail stretching several times each day to avoid inflexibility. "Early and often" is the secret slogan toward normalcy.

Stretching: A week or two after breast surgery, letting warm waters shower against your scars will help them soften enough to increase your arm-stretching exercises. Remember to continue them well into your recovery days. In order to be as physically agile as possible, consider taking massages and physical therapy, especially if you develop pain in either skin or tight muscles during your post-treatment days.

EYEBROWS & EYELASHES

When you find that your eyebrows and lashes have evaporated into thin air, locate your normal arch and then use either brush-on eye make-up or an eyebrow pencil to match your natural hair color. Make each eyebrow fuller around the nose, then gradually thin the line out as you go toward the outside of the arch. With practice you can do wonders. As for the lashes, your eyeliner or a soft eyebrow pencil can be drawn above and below your eyes where lashes will grow again. Just a line will help your eyes give the impression of growing lashes. Go easy so you don't end up looking like Spot, the dog with one black eye!

EYES

Blurred vision: Rarely do patients experience blurred or diminished eyesight. You don't need to be overly concerned; but if this does occur, you must report it to your medical team. They will know just what to do to correct it.

Commercial tears: Unlike your nose, your eyes may become dry, especially while you sleep. Using commercial tears should help solve the problem until your own tear ducts and glands recuperate enough to do their job again.

Vitamins: The vitamins that are especially good for your eyes are vitamins A, C, and E. Remember ACE = Always Clear Eyes. Small amounts of zinc are also considered to be advantageous. Many multiple vitamins contain these ingredients, but you should check with an ophthalmologist before prescribing them for yourself.

Wet: Treatment sometimes can affect your eyes by making them too wet. Only a fresh soft handkerchief will help this condition. The sad movies or poignant moments may still cause natural tears to flow as they always have.

FOOD

Bacteria: Raw eggs and raw meat may contain harmful bacteria, so be sure all such dishes continue to cook long enough after other ingredients are added. Sandwich spreads and salads are ideal places to add hard-boiled eggs, thus sneaking extra nutrients into your diet.

Bananas: A favorite saying of everyone once was "An apple a day keeps the doctor away." That may still be true since all fruits help balance our bodily needs. Today, however, the banana is threatening to usurp the fruit throne. When very few things appeal to you, a slice of a banana will be rather easy to swallow. It contains sucrose and fructose plus fiber, thus giving you a snack and an instant boost of energy.

Bland — Attempt to eat: The more bland and moist your food is, the easier you will find it is to swallow on "bad" days. When nothing appeals to your taste buds, you still must attempt to eat something. Even breaking toast, crackers, gingersnaps, etc., into finger-sized bits may be worth a try.

Bland — Try these: When nothing else sounds possible to eat, try applesauce or egg custard. Some people can eat cups of flavored gelatin, but the flavors seem too strong and too artificial for many people.

Blenders: Blenders can be among your best friends. They allow many nutritious drinks to be made quickly. Drinks are readily digestible and slide down with ease. Also they are generally cold, which is more acceptable to most people than many hot things seem to be, often even including coffee. You might consider having iced coffee with a scoop of ice cream.

Boost or Ensure: When your appetite is gone and your energy is like a damp washcloth, try drinks like "Boost" or "Ensure." They come in many flavors and quickly supply you with the nutrients you need.

Bran & fruit: As your ability to eat returns, raisin bran cereal, with a handful of bran buds and fresh fruit mixed in, tastes much better than prune juice! It's good for you in unspeakable ways.

Calories & cheese, two hints for maintaining weight:

+ Calories can be increased for reluctant eaters by folding a bit of whipped cream into vegetable purees, mashed potatoes, pancakes, waffles, puddings, gelatins, and even atop cups of hot chocolate or coffee.

+ Cheese melted on almost any vegetable, sandwich, omelet, biscuit, or casserole also will help add calories when you aren't eating enough.

Cereals: Things that slip down your throat with ease are much more appealing than foods that need to be chewed. One exception is Cheerios-type cereals, because they become soft after the first crunching bite. When your food makes a chomping sound, you feel as if you are really eating again.

Cottage cheese: Cottage cheese makes an easy trip to the stomach and can be mixed with fruit or other chopped foods of your choice.

Dried fruit: Dried fruits such as raisins, figs, dates, apricots, and prunes make nice snacks or breakfast food, and even desserts, especially if you cook them a bit. They help increase calories when added to muffins, bran cereals, cakes, vegetables, or anything else you can also think of baking. Incidentally, canned and frozen vegetables plus fruit have been shown to be as nutritious as the fresh kind and are often less expensive to boot.

Easy & Nutritions: Some foods slide down easily, even when the flavor seems reduced. People with dulled taste buds and upset stomachs can usually manage the nutritious foods listed here:

+Applesauce
+Apple Juice (diluted)
+Bananas
+Boost or Ensure (cold)
+Canned baby carrots
+Canned peaches & pears
+Cottage cheese
+Egg custard
+Egg salad (*even a sliver of shell might gag you*)
+Eggs any style
+Ginger Tea (in sips)
+Mashed potatoes
+Oatmeal
+Pastas
+Popsicles
+Scrambled & soft boiled eggs
+Seedless grapes
+Toast (in tiny bits mixed with eggs, applesauce, or anything wet)
+Watermelon
+Yogurt (plain or frozen)

Experiment — Add moisture - Meats:
+ Protein rich meats, while important to your diet, are often as tasteless as cardboard during mealtimes. The moisture of applesauce used as a topping makes meat much more palatable.

Experiment — Add moisture - More items:
+ Using sauces or gravy on dry food will add moisture to many protein-providing meals, especially for patients who have trouble swallowing.
+ Cheese, eggs, and milk also may be used on any of the following: meatloaf, casseroles, mashed potatoes, quiches, puddings and custards.
+ For acquiring extra protein, you may include ice cream or yogurt.

These foods may be eaten as they are or added to beverages, atop fruit, pies, cereals, and even between cookies or cake slices. Try your hand at being creatively inventive.

Experiment — Crunchy toppings: Nuts, wheat germ, and seeds can be added to casseroles, muffins, waffles, pancakes, and cookies or sprinkled on cereal, ice cream, fruit, salads, and desserts as a crunchy topping. Sometimes you could even roll them onto bananas or blend them into sauces. All the protein you can eat will benefit your recovery in tasty ways.

Experiment — Suggestions from others: Be willing to try any food that friends, family or other patients suggest. We all take individually prescribed treatments and may respond in ways different from other people. Actually, some foods that seem intolerable to you after one treatment frequently will taste okay after a later treatment.

Ginger cookies: Moravian ginger cookies are very thin – thin enough not to turn into clay in your mouth when nibbled. The ginger helps tranquilize nausea.

Ginger tea: During your "better" days, even before your stomach begins to feel upset, a quick snack with a sip or two of ginger tea may help.

Meals on wheels: "Meals on Wheels" is an option available in many communities. Especially if you live alone, this service will supply nutritious food that may last you for several meals. You might eat only small amounts, but will probably enjoy food more when it's prepared by someone else.

Munching: Munching food slowly while reading, watching TV, or visiting with other people could help take your mind off the snack or meal and allow you to eat more. It is imperative to maintain your weight as much as possible.

Nutritious: Living on ice cream and Chinese egg drop soup for a few days or more isn't that bad.

Offers of food: If friends offer to cook and bring you food, tell them you would love that. Don't hesitate to accept any offerings, especially if you have someone else who can be spared a cooking chore. It wouldn't hurt to tell them what sort of things you *can* eat. They will appreciate your suggestions.

Peanut butter: Blending peanut butter with milk or ice cream is another way to add needed proteins to your diet. It has been written that Elvis Presley's favorite was a banana and peanut butter sandwich mixed with a small amount of mayonnaise. This has always been a great treat for children in the Deep South.

Popsicles & watermelons: Popsicles and watermelons aren't very nourishing, but they are moist, cold, and tasty to the palate when most other things are less appealing.

Prunes: Need a glass of prune juice? Try it warm for an added effect. Some people feel that it can be improved when mixed with one-eighth cup of grape juice. Elimination problems during your cancer battle can be lessened with daily help.

Raw — Never: You should never eat raw vegetables until you have finished taking chemotherapy. Then gradually experiment with carrots, cucumbers, celery, or cauliflower by trying a children's long-time tradition of using peanut butter as a raw vegetable dip. Yummy! The smooth rather than crunchy variety of peanut butter is preferred, and mixing it with small amounts of mayonnaise makes it easier to dip and spread.

Recipe (my doctor approved it for me): If you aren't feeling hungry but know that you need nourishment, try this doctor's recipe:

8 oz. chilled Gatorade

2 or 3 oz. half-and-half from the dairy counter

1 raw egg

Mix thoroughly in a blender and drink, unless you are afraid of raw eggs. These ingredients are good and good for you.

Red meat: Red meat is likely to taste and smell stronger and less appealing during cancer treatment. Dairy products, finely diced turkey or chicken, mild-tasting fish, and meat substitutes like eggs and cheese may suit your taste buds better. Sometimes marinating chicken or fish in fruit juices or sweet-and-sour sauces may help. Adding meat and vegetables to broth or creamy soups could be another way of getting nutritious meals into your system.

Servings per day: If you add fruit to your cereal and have a glass of juice at breakfast, add lettuce and tomato to your sandwich at lunch, and have a salad with one cooked vegetable for dinner, then you will find that you have eaten at least the recommended five servings per day.

Soups: Soups and broths sit well on tummies that need to be treated gently.

Sugar substitute: Always check the labels of sugar-free foods. Be aware that many sugar substitutes contain sorbitol, which may cause diarrhea in some people.

Taste — Metallic or paper: When everything tastes either metallic or like paper, snacking every three or four hours can usually avoid the queasies and modify your taste buds. Any food you can sneak into your stomach will help you perk up a bit. Make a list of nutritious foods that appeal to you.

Tea: Alkylamines which are found in tea seem to boost some of the most important immune cells in the human body. Called "gamma-delta T cells," they attack germs. Smaller concentrations of Alkylamines are located in some mushrooms, apples, and wines. The same kinds of immune responses are important in fighting cancer. Isn't it worth drinking more tea, eating more apples and mushrooms, and drinking a little wine? You bet!

Upset tummy: Try eating oatmeal or drinking sips of ginger tea to help calm your upset stomach.

Veggies & fruit: The American Cancer Society guidelines on nutrition and physical activity for cancer protection suggest that Mom was right when she told you to eat your vegetables. Generally the more colorful fruits and vegetables have the most nutrients to keep you healthy.

Veggies well-cooked: Be sure that all of your vegetables are well cooked for the duration of your chemotherapy. Because they are soft, they will be easier to swallow. Even during the first five "bad" days after your treatments, cooked carrots, cauliflower, broccoli, and green beans taste much like "real food." No meat seems to fit this description.

Vitamins: As a safeguard, you may want to add a multi-vitamin each day to your breakfast menu. Ask your doctor which one is best for you.

FORGIVENESS

Some friends may avoid being with you just because they care for you and don't quite know what to say. Forgive their hesitation based on fear for their own vulnerability and for their reaction to your illness. The very word *cancer* frightens some people just the way the mention of snakes or spiders may do to others. Once they hear that your outlook is positive, they are more likely to call or visit.

FREE BRASSIERE

Some lingerie specialty shops have custom-designed brassieres for cancer patients and Medicare will pay for them. You might make some phone calls to discover if any such shops in your area offer this benefit.

GOALS TO ANTICIPATE

Make a written list of some of the things you can look forward to enjoying or accomplishing during your "best" days. If your chemo treatments are a standard 21 days apart, there will be at least as many "best" days as "bad" and "better" ones. Even light housework and grocery shopping will give you goals to anticipate with pleasure because they were ordinary activities before you became ill.

GRAB BARS

When showering, it is wise to use grab bars. They will steady you as you enter the stall or tub and help if you become dizzy while bending over to retrieve slippery soap.

GROANS

It is a known fact that deep sighs and groaning when your body aches will help you get through the rough   times. Allow yourself these small compensations, especially when you are alone.

HAIR

Bald — Careful wishes: Be careful for the things you wish would happen in your life. With your hair all gone, your secret wish to become a movie star may have come true. You just didn't expect that you might be asked to play an alien!

Bald — Cold head: Having no hair will mean having a cold head in winter if you sleep and walk around without headgear, which can be found in any cancer center.

Bald — Shampoo: Make sure to shampoo your bald head, wash your neck and behind your ears, just as you were taught years ago.

Cut early: Scalp hair appearing on your shoulders is a strong signal that it is time to have your hair cut very short. Early haircuts look rather chic. Many women even have their scalps shaved once the extreme loss begins. Psychologically it is much less distressing to lose short hair than large unshorn clumps.

Departed: Probably it will surprise you how disturbing the loss of hair can be. We all want to look as attractive as possible and hair is more important than anyone thinks it will be. Ah, well [sigh]. Wigs, caps, and bandanas come to the rescue until the newer sprouts appear about six to eight weeks after the end of treatments. Remember: for everything there is a season!

Facial: Unfair! Wild facial hairs which were simply annoying before cancer treatments, are among the very first hairs to return when treatments end and new hair begins to grow again.

Lashes: If you lose your hair, chances are that you will also lose your eyelashes. Without them your eyes may feel strangely different and sometimes quite dry, requiring eye drops.

Legs: Hairless legs are so smooth that when you sleep on your side, one leg will probably slide right off the other! Pajamas can remedy this odd problem.

Nightcap: For women with little or no hair, one nighttime comfort in chilly weather or in an air-conditioned room is being able to pull a soft nightcap down over your eyes and enter into a warm, dark hole of comfort.

Nose: No one ever thinks to mention that hair disappears from inside your nose! Whatever the reason for this, you'll have a leaking faucet much of the time. Be prepared or be embarrassed.

Wigs: Should you choose to buy a wig, your doctor may write a prescription for you. Payment by Medicare will be accepted without any question. In fact, reputable wig shops will even do the paperwork for you. If you are not yet eligible for Medicare, check with your insurance agent; many insurance companies may also pick up that cost.

HEARING LOSS

If you notice a hearing loss during treatment, tell your doctor. It could be caused by one of your medications or something as simple as wax buildup.

HOT FLASHES

An action triggered by hormonal changes due to decreased estrogen levels can cause hot flashes, which may result in the opening and closing of blood vessels. Consequently, some women may experience these hot flashes during their treatment days.

INFECTIONS

Be aware that you are more susceptible than ever to infections during cancer treatments, so wash your hands many times a day with bacteria-fighting brand soaps such as Dial.

INSURANCE

If you are ever uncomfortable with any part of your treatment, ask questions and don't be afraid to get a second opinion. See if your insurance policy will pay for an appointment with another doctor.

JEWELRY

Be sure to remove rings and any other jewelry before edema causes them to become too tight or weight loss makes them too loose due to dehydration.

JOKES

Realize that on some days, no jokes will seem the least bit funny. If it's a printed joke such as E-mail brings, try saving the forwards until you feel better and you'll be amazed at how much improved the joke will become. The same joke that brought a groan on a bad day may even make you laugh aloud when the timing is right.

LACTOSE INTOLERANCE

Normal aging results in a lower lactase production. The inability to digest the sugar in dairy products can cause diarrhea, bloating, and gas. The trouble is due to a lack of the enzyme lactase in the small intestine. Chemo requires the use of toxic chemicals, thereby causing further aggravation.

MAMMOGRAMS — SPREAD THE WORD

Many people will ask if it is okay to tell others about your health. Consider your feelings about privacy and decide whether or not you want to have the word spread. This would be a great time to suggest that they encourage others to get regular mammograms and stress the importance of these precautions to everyone.

MEMORY ET CETERA

Chemo treatments may temporarily aggravate your short-term memory and other cognitive functions, thereby causing problems with quick thinking, organization, focusing, and the inability to do two things at once. Keep notes within easy reach and you will become less frustrated. This annoying side effect is generally referred to as *chemobrain*.

MEN AS NURSES

Women, don't blame your man too much if he is a poor nurse. Although men with training in the medical field can be excellent nurses, most males were not reared to be caregivers. Many husbands see things differently from their wives; they want to fix problems and protect other people from danger. When they can't, they feel helpless and tend to become frustrated, angry, or guilty. When they ask what they can do for you, suggest some small thing. It will ease their desire to show you their complete and continuing support.

MOUTH

Bad taste: Nearly everyone taking cancer treatments complains of bad tastes, especially after eating. To help alleviate this problem, some people like to suck cinnamon "red hots" or other hard candies. Teeth beware!

Dentures: If you wear removable dentures, you might find that your gums are extra tender or swollen. You may be told to discontinue wearing the dentures until your radiation therapy has ended. Gum sores are also a problem with chemotherapy, so be particularly careful about infections because during this time your mouth will heal very slowly.

Dry: Dry mouth is a term used when your mouth seems to be perpetually parched. This seems like an odd term, but if you happen to have this side effect, you'll know that just saying you are thirsty is an understatement. You will appreciate the importance of drinking large amounts of water to keep from being dehydrated.

Dry — Glycerin: Pharmacists have suggested that applying a small amount of glycerin to your lips will bring relief before surgery to patients suffering from excessively dry mouths or cracked lips. Glycerin, a slightly yellow liquid, is a rather sweet moisturizer that can be purchased in small, reasonably priced bottles at most pharmacies. You will also appreciate its use if you are recovering from surgery or at any time when you are temporarily not allowed to drink water or other liquids. If given by a caregiver, this welcomed glycerin may easily be applied by using cotton swabs such as Q-tips.

Floss & water pick usage: Gently using waxed non-shredding dental floss to protect your tender gums could help reduce some of the unpleasant taste in your mouth. A water pick is another dentist-approved instrument that aids in maintaining healthy gums.

Fresheners: Some people have discovered that Listerine's "PocketPac" dissolvable strips help bad-tasting mouths feel cleaner. Sucking peppermint pinwheels or any other hard candies may help "dragon breath" disappear. Chewing gum also may work briefly.

Petroleum jelly: Using petroleum jelly will help your lips feel better when they become dry or sore.

Plastic utensils: Eating with plastic instead of metal and silver utensils lessens metallic aftertastes.

Salt: When treatments start, use salt water for oral rinses at the first sign of discomfort. Often they can help keep sores from developing into a problem.

Sores: Sores in the mouth and throat can be aggravated by citrus and spicy foods. Gargling with a glass of warm salt water may bring wonderful relief.

Teeth & tongue: Frequent brushing of your teeth and tongue can be quite helpful in controlling that awful taste that seems to haunt the mouths of most patients. Baking soda may help to refresh your mouth while neutralizing any acids that can hurt your teeth.

Teeth — Use soft brush: Using a soft toothbrush more often than just after meals and at bedtime is a suggestion for folks who may have become unusually susceptible to mouth infections.

MUSIC

Easy listening music soothes the spirit. The relaxation that it offers is especially helpful during difficult mealtimes.

NAILS

Avoid infections: If you frequently wash clothing or dishes, have a hand cream nearby and use it often or wear rubber gloves to avoid infections.

Manicures: If you have a good manicurist, make clear to her that she must be extremely careful of the hand closest to your surgery. Your cuticle must be pushed very gently and never cut at all. By being specific, you will be doing a favor to both her and her future cancer customers. As such a patient, you may want to explain that most arm infections begin in the hands and nails.

Massaging: Massage cuticles with a cream to prevent dryness, splitting, tearing, or hangnails. Dry nails tend to weaken, and fungus infections easily can invade nail beds.

No pain: If your nails become discolored, you'll find that there is no pain involved. Actually nails seem to grow faster and stronger during treatments.

Polish: Wait to use nail polish and artificial nails until after all cancer treatment is completed.

NOSE

Body odor: Physicians will assure you that only you can smell your own chemically-induced body odors. Your nose sensitivity will be far greater than that of non-patients.

Cold: Despite the weather, some people find that their noses are always cold; a heating pad should work just fine.

Handkerchief: Always have a hankie nearby. It is needed not only for sinus drainage; it can also be a great mask when strong perfumes or other odors become obnoxious. This is true especially when you are riding in an enclosed space such as an automobile or elevator.

Odors: our sense of smell during your "bad" days will be very acute and many things will be bothersome; unfortunately, among the worst is food being cooked for other members in your home. Even before someone starts cooking, closing the doors between yourself and the kitchen will help quite a bit.

Pets: If you own house pets, expect to be bothered by their odors. Giving them more frequent baths helps very little, unfortunately. Of course, you can buy an electric odor ender if you can spare $400 [Ouch!]. There is one on the market; it's a metal tower called Ionic Breeze and works very well. It will diminish the smells immensely - or you can send your pets on a six month vacation *anywhere* else.

Sensitivity: Perfumes, bath oils, face powders and other powders should never be used during your treatment. They all may bother sensitive noses and may even affect treatment effectiveness as well. People visiting or taking care of you also need to avoid using perfume since your sense of smell is so acute.

NOSEBLEEDS

Are you one of those chemo patients who tend to suffer from nosebleeds? Nasal strips sold to prevent snoring may also aid your breathing if the bleeding causes you to have an uncomfortable overnight accumulation of blood. They certainly would be worth consideration.

OVERPROTECTION

You will enjoy friends showing concern for you, no matter how sleepy or sick you are. Honestly, patients may sleep at anytime, night or day. If your family tends to overprotect you by asking friends not to phone, you could feel that no one really cares. Those who call, even if you feel too ill to talk directly to them, can be handled by your answering machine or someone else who is taking messages for you. Knowing that people are thinking of you means everything.

PAMPER

Allow your friends and family to pamper you a bit. It makes them feel that they are needed and a part of your recovery. They are!

PETS

Need attention: Pets sense that you are not well and will try to comfort you. Allow them to do so if you can. They need attention because they cannot comprehend why you are unwilling to pet or play with them.

Sympathetic: When you are extremely ill and feel guilty about having to neglect your pets' attempts to show their love, remember that they are more forgiving and sympathetic than most people. They will forget and forgive all past slights.

PHLEGM

The secretions of thick, stringy mucus of the respiratory tract that annoy everyone during heavy colds must be tolerated by many people during cancer treatments. Isolating yourself from crowds during flu season should help reduce the development of contagious infections. Phlegm irritation often lingers long after you think colds have left your body, but your throat knows that some evil threat is still in the vicinity.

PILLS VS. EMPTY STOMACH

One practice to avoid is taking pills on a totally empty stomach unless your doctor or prescription directions specifically tell you to do so.

PLAY — NOT TODAY

Sometimes you must tell youngsters, "I'm sorry, but I just can't play today."

PRETEND

Try being an actor. Surely you can pretend to feel better than you actually do for the short time you are with other patients. It is remarkable how contagious even mock cheerfulness can be. Soon you and everyone else should be in better spirits.

PURSE

One way to protect your surgery arm is to form the habit of carrying your handbag in your other hand or over your other shoulder.

PUT FORTH EFFORT QUOTE

We are free agents to be whatever we decided we want to be as long as we believe it is possible and are willing to put in the effort and discipline necessary to bring it about. Thea Alexander "2150 AD, A Novel"

RESTLESS LEGS SYNDROME (RLS)

Aches & pains: Cancer medications may be a cause of restless legs at night. Be sure to mention any leg pains and involuntary twitching or throbbing sensations to your doctor. Getting out of bed and walking around a bit seems to still them for a while. You might want to try lying on your tummy with a pillow under the lower part of your stomach for about five minutes.

True or false: Perhaps this is only an old wives' tale, but some people guarantee the success of placing a large bar of soap under the bottom sheet of RLS sufferers while they sleep. They claim that this remedy will reduce the problem considerably. For some unknown reason, all brands don't seem to work for this purpose. Incidentally, one newspaper column has letters from several readers saying that soap also works for nighttime leg cramps. You can bet that sufferers and their bed partners will at least be willing to give this a try. Sometimes it seems that truth is indeed stranger than fiction.

SHY

When you first enter a group of fellow patients, don't be shy. Introduce yourself and you'll find you share many things in common, paving the way for friendships and support, both given and received.

SIGHS

Sometimes deep sighs actually can alleviate pains in the lining of your lungs.

SKIN

Bra straps & other clothing: If your bra straps rub your shoulders during your radiation phase, they can increase the risk of cutting into your extremely tender skin. Loose clothes will be safer and more comfortable. You may want to try cotton camisoles which are found in lingerie departments. If you want to save your dresses and shirts from ink stains caused by your radiation markings, remove your bra altogether. In its place, consider wearing men's cotton undershirts beneath your outer clothing. Wearing a man's size that fits you rather tightly should give you some breast support.

Care: Care of your skin is very important with radiation therapy. When washing your treatment areas, use lukewarm water and very mild soaps such as Dove or Ivory. Bathe and dry your affected skin gently. Be sure not to use any bath oils, talcum powder, or perfumes. Some ointments and even prescription medications may worsen the condition of your skin.

Care & caution: There are many prohibitive rules because your skin is so fragile that it might crack and become moist. Use ointments only after any treatment that day is completed and only if you are certain that there are no breaks in your skin. Always check questionable products with someone on your radiation team. Most 95-100% pure aloe gels that are acquired from a druggist or are cut directly from a growing plant may be used at bedtime.

Cotton: During radiation treatment and continuing through the time your skin begins to heal, plan to wear soft cotton clothing. This is not the time for nylon or synthetics which bind or cling easily since they may irritate and cause pain to your fragile skin.

Dermatologist: Paget's disease is a rare form of breast cancer. If you are already seeing a dermatologist who inspects your skin closely for any pre-cancers on your chest, you will be alerted of any signs of this disease in its earliest stages.

Dry: Unusually dry skin is often experienced during chemotherapy and radiation. Using mild anti-bacterial soaps and lukewarm showers plus lotions containing moisturizers should help considerably. Be sure to avoid hormone creams containing hydrocortisone as they may slow down the immune system.

Face: If you have increased sensitivity to various face creams that used to serve you well before treatments, try switching to Vaseline and leave the cosmetic makeup in the drawer for a while.

Fringes: Would you believe that skin can form fringes on your heels? If they do happen to develop, try using a pumice stone. Our bodies replace dead skin the same way they do dead hair. Buying your stone early and using it during your showers may save you from developing these *tassels.*

Healing: Polysporin heals cuts and open sores while warding off infections on thin dry skin, and Dial soap has been recommended to me for use as the preferred skin cleanser after surgery.

Ointments: Avoid any damage to your now extremely fragile skin. This includes sun rays. Protect yourself with moisturizer ointments and insect repellents. Infections heal more slowly now than they did before chemotherapy or radiation treatments began.

Razor: All oncologists remind patients to use only electric razors during and after treatments; this is especially important when the platelet count is low. When cancer treatment ends, skin is extremely thin and may be nicked, causing you to bleed easily until your body readjusts. After your hair begins growing back, be sure that you continue to use an electric razor when shaving your legs and underarms.

SPF 15: Always stay away from prolonged sun exposure and use sunscreen with SPF 15 or higher.

Steroids: Some steroids given to combat side effects may cause a rash. Your doctor may prescribe Benzoyl Peroxide Gel 10%, which has been known to help ease rashes.

Trick: Remember how sensitive your scalp becomes whenever you develop a high fever? It hurts! Losing your hair feels about the same way. A trick that may help reduce the sensitivity is to make an ice pack. How? Use your freezer to form a cap by placing a wet washcloth over an upside-down bowl about the size of your head. After a short time, remove the frozen cloth and try it on for size and comfort. It will become a perfect temporary ice cap.

Wigs: Treatments may change your skin coloring dramatically. Expect it and enjoy the variety. It could mean that you will want to wear clothing you would normally avoid. The fun comes in wearing different colored wigs which will look great. You can be a blonde one day and a redhead the next. Wigs come in various styles as well as colors, so you might as well have some fun playing dress-up.

SLEEP

Sandman: While coaxing the sandman to visit, a warm bathrobe may serve you well through chills and middle-of-the-night prowls. You will find that there is much comfort in cuddling with your favorite robe and a soft blanket.

Television: If you suddenly awaken in the middle of the night while watching a late television show after finally falling asleep, flip off the TV, and head for your bed before you become fully alert. There's a good chance that you may go right back to sleep.

SLIPPING MEMORY

Ask your oncologist if vitamins C and B12 are okay in combination with your treatment chemicals. It is said that these vitamins help short term memory loss due to chemotherapy. If you don't want to try this remedy, just wait it out and gradually your memory *will* improve.

SLOW DOWN

It is okay if you have to do things more slowly or less perfectly than before treatments. It's also okay if you are on an outing and need to return home earlier than you had planned. Your main job of the moment is getting rid of the disease itself, and your body will dictate to you when you have done enough for one day.

VERY LOW BLOOD PRESSURE

Dizziness is one sign that your blood pressure has dropped to a very low reading. Of course you should mention it to your health team members; but a quick fix is chicken soup, Gatorade or, believe it or not, potato chips! Salt on the chips is the miracle worker that should come to your aid.

WALK DON'T RUN

On your "best" days continue to *walk* while your energy level is highest; don't run, not even to answer the door bell or telephone. The last thing you need is to invite injuries or bruises.

WATER

Bottled: Always remember to keep a bottle of water handy; sometimes you'll prefer it cold, other times at room temperature.

Clips: Carrying your friendly water bottle around with you is now in style. There are even plastic clips that you can attach to a belt or to the window of your car to encourage an even stronger relationship with your "liquid companion."

Exercises: A week or two after surgery, letting warm water cascade against your scars will soften the skin. Just do a few stretch exercises right in the shower while clinging to a hand bar so as not to lose your balance.

Use a straw: It is said that sipping water and other fluids through a straw can trick you into drinking more than normal. Another hint is that anything tastes better when it is drunk from a stemmed glass or, better still, from a *crystal* stemmed glass.

WEAR — NOT THESE

Women, take heed: forget about wearing heels that may make you totter, jeans so tight that breathing becomes difficult, and skirts that are too short for you to sit down without worrying about "southern exposure." At least recover from cancer before becoming a fashion plate!

WEIGHT

Don't diet: Certain anticancer drugs cause body fluids to build up excessively. Since many folks lose weight during treatment, it is very important that you *do not diet* before talking with your doctor. It may even be wise for you to check with a dietitian. Keep in mind that the American Cancer Society offers many free services. That's where some of your donations have gone all these years.

Gain: Gaining weight may occur with some cancer programs. If it is necessary to life as you prefer to live it, you can buy larger clothes to be comfortable and concentrate on regaining your health without even getting on the scales until after your cancer journey has come to an end.

Idea: As your weight changes from thick to thin or vice versa, consider buying a few basic slacks with elastic waist bands. They will see you through your cancer treatments with much more comfort and less need for constant shopping sprees, when you least want to buy new clothes.

Loss — Eat anyway: If losing weight has always been one of your dreams, you'll probably feel fine about pounds melting away; but during cancer treatments isn't a wise time to lose intentionally. You are extremely vulnerable to infections and anemia. Force yourself to eat and maintain your weight until you finish all treatments. Anyway, you'll probably lose plenty without trying.

Loss — Liquids: Eating and drinking lots of water and supplementary drinks (such as Boost Plus, Carnation Instant Breakfast, and Ensure) will keep you from losing so much weight. It is very important not to lose too much at once, thereby becoming weak. Malnutrition can make problems like anemia worsen, and of course a weakened immune system invites infection.

WHY ASPIRIN

According to current studies by research scientists, a daily ingestion of baby aspirin (81 mg.) seems to lessen the chance of hormone-dependent breast cancers in women. Check with your health team to determine if it may be right for you.

WIGS

In public: Wearing wigs in public can make you feel more like your old self, but they may become hot and bothersome. Around home you will probably just choose to leave them off in summer and then switch to a soft cap in cooler weather.

Mirror: After the initial shock of viewing your bald head, there is something not that bad about seeing yourself in the mirror. It is easier to care for a bald scalp than for hair that won't do as you wish! Slip on a wig or hat and you're ready to greet the world.

Paper caps: Some creative women have found that paper coffee filters serve well as inner caps under their wigs. The filters are absorbent and keep scalps from itching or becoming tacky in warm weather.

Skull cap: When wearing a wig, you'll find that a cotton skull cap or bandana will protect your head from feeling overly hot or sticky. The Harley-

Davidson type under your wig does a good job. Just flip the ties and the bandana tail inside to develop a small knot so your wig will be better anchored.

Uplifting: When ladies make an effort to wear lipstick and a wig or a new hat, they usually find that they actually feel better and it might even make other patients also want to dress up a bit. A little vanity goes a long way toward uplifting spirits.

WORDS

Acceptable: Most patients are very open in their discussions, whether talking with men or women. They freely use words like bowel movement or BM, urine, diarrhea, breasts, prostate, or anything else that needs to be said. Everything is acceptable and no one seems prudish or embarrassed. Everyone learns from the comments and experiences of others.

Be careful: Think before expressing yourself too openly to other patients. One can never be sure if the spoken words today will later become memories of dread and despair to another.

Silence: Be very sensitive in choosing your words and moments when you speak with other patients. Looking them straight in the eyes will give you a good clue as to how they are feeling about your subject matter. Many times silence is more healing than conversation, except of course when it's good news from your doctor.

YOU SHOULD KNOW

Cancer develops for unknown reasons. Nothing you have ever done in your life has caused you to have breast cancer. It is caused by neither stress nor injury to the breast, and is not contagious. Furthermore, many women who develop cancer don't even have a known history of the disease in their families. So don't ever feel guilty.

YOU SHOULD TALK TO SOMEONE

If you have a male oncologist and feel comfortable with him, you should be able to chat about your present concerns. Tell him about anything that disturbs you, whether they are sexual questions, doubts about the ability to complete the prescribed treatments, hormonal changes, or fears of death. If you would prefer to speak with a female doctor or nurse, select one with whom you have established a rapport and ask her if you and she could have a woman to woman conversation. She will have answers to your questions or know where to find them.

YOUR HEALTH SAFEGUARD

As a precaution, never have your surgery arm used for any blood samples or blood pressure, but consider wearing one of the metallic medical alert bracelets. If you are in an accident and can't communicate with the emergency crew, they will be aware of your bracelet and act accordingly.

YOUR PORT — PROTECTION

If you have a port under your left collarbone and are still driving a car, you may feel much more comfortable if you purchase a soft padded cover for your seat belt since the belt must cross directly over your port. When you are the passenger and your port is located on your *right* side, this same protection will be effective.

YOUR PORT — REMOVAL DATE

When your chemotherapy days have ended, you may be overeager to have your port removed at once. Physicians won't be in such a hurry. They need to check your progress for a while to assure more treatments are not required. Although people seldom need their ports to remain for very long, keeping them in place for a time is wise; once they are removed, a second surgery would be required. The port is neither unsightly nor painful, so don't rush things.

YOUR VEGETABLES & FRUITS

Most people won't heed this tip, but it must be mentioned. Because your immune system is very vulnerable right now, you must be extra careful of fruit from third world countries where their health standards are often less strict than those in the United States. Realizing this, it might be prudent to rinse and soak your vegetables and fruit with a teaspoon of baking soda mixed in a cup of water. It will take just a few moments and is another way to protect your fragile state of health.

Chapter 10

General Information

BEGINNINGS

Be prepared: If for any reason you need to see a new doctor, you probably will be required to produce former mammogram and ultrasound films, biopsy slides, and pathology reports for comparison with future procedures. Having the addresses and phone numbers of former doctors on hand, plus any insurance cards, will speed the preliminary process of becoming a new patient. Each specialist also will ask for your medical history, including the dosage of medications that you are currently taking. Being prepared to produce these records will save you return visits or phone calls.

Documents:
+ Advance Directives
+ Designation of a Health Care Surrogate
+ Health Care Durable Power of Attorney
+ Insurance Information
+ Living Will
+ Permission for Organ/Tissue Donation

If you have already prepared the documents, take them with you on surgery day. Include phone numbers and addresses. Even with them in hand, you will be required to sign a disclaimer. If you have none of these documents, you still may be treated without them. Nevertheless, now probably would be a good time to take care of this matter as you prepare for surgery.

Insurance: A wise decision would be to contact your health insurance carrier to review your health plan, preferably before any treatment begins.

Stages of breast cancer:
+ Stages I and II are early stages of breast cancer.
+ Stage I means that the tumor is about one inch across and cancer cells are less likely to have spread beyond the breast.
+ Stage II means that the tumor is less than one inch across but the cancer has spread to the lymph nodes under the arm; or the tumor is between one and two inches, with or without underarm

nodes affected; or the tumor is larger than two inches, but has not spread to the underarm lymph nodes.

+ Stage III is called locally advanced cancer. The tumor is more than two inches across and has spread to the underarm lymph nodes; or the cancer is extensive in the underarm lymph nodes; or the cancer has spread to the lymph nodes near the breastbone or to other tissues near the breast.

+ Stage IV is metastatic cancer which has spread beyond the breast and underarm lymph nodes to other parts of the body. Women in this stage may have surgery or radiation therapy to control the cancer in the breast. Radiation may also be useful to control tumors in other parts of the body. Although cancer cells may metastasize through the blood or lymphatic system in any stage, it is extremely rare in the earlier stages.

Types of surgery: There are two types of surgery for breast cancer. One, a lumpectomy, is called breast-conserving surgery because only part of the breast is removed. The other, a mastectomy, involves removing the entire breast; however, there are many types of mastectomies which your physician will gladly explain.

Types of treatment: The main types of treatment for breast cancer are:

+ Surgery to remove the primary tumor and contiguous cancer cells
+ Radiation therapy that uses high-energy rays to kill cancer cells
+ Chemotherapy that uses drugs to kill cancer cells
+ Therapy that uses hormone-type drugs to stop the growth of cancer cells

All four are essential to some stages of breast cancer, but an early stage diagnosis often effectively requires only surgery and/or radiation.

MISCELLANEOUS

Alcohol & tobacco — Dramatic: It has been proven that people who use alcohol and tobacco together are at a greater risk of having cancer than those who smoke or drink without combining the two. The risk of breast cancer seems dramatically to affect women who drink alcohol, increasing their susceptibility to infections due to a low white blood count. Of course tobacco creates a threat of lung cancer in both men and women.

Alcohol & tobacco — Risks: It has been reported that the consumption of more than two alcoholic drinks per day can, in both men and women, heighten the possibility of cancer in the areas of the mouth, esophagus, pharynx, larynx and liver. Both alcohol and tobacco affect the immune system. When they are used at the same time, the risk of developing these cancers increases even more than when one is drinking and not smoking or vice versa.

Anorexia: Although you may be pleased with many lost pounds, don't allow yourself to fall into the trap of liking the slim look so much that you are unhealthy and look frail rather than just thin. You will always have a tummy and some loose flesh. That is the same trap that snags some teenagers into dissatisfaction with their bodies. You could develop anorexia nervosa, a serious nervous disorder in eating behavior marked especially by a pathological fear of any weight gain. This condition leads to faulty eating patterns, malnutrition, and unusually excessive weight loss. Most people are more critical of their own bodies than of yours! The truth is that your persona, not your body, is the most attractive thing about you.

Appointments: — Delays: Always expect some appointment delays in seeing your doctors and nurses. Patience really helps everyone. Use the waiting time to share experiences with other detained patients. Friends are easily made in cancer clinics. Every patient understands what other patients are going through more thoroughly than anyone else, including most of the doctors themselves.

Appointments: — Dentist: While you are being treated, consult your oncologist for advice regarding the timing of any dental appointment, including professional cleaning. Especially now, your mouth and gums are exceedingly sensitive and prone to bleeding and infections. If an emergency occurs, ask about the need for antibiotics.

Appointments: — More than one: Some cancer patients need more than one treatment per day. If that is recommended for you, accept the expert opinion of your doctor and cooperate fully.

Appointments: — Never skip: No matter how ill you feel, try never to skip any of your scheduled chemo treatments, Neupogen injections, or radiation procedures. Timing for each step of the way has been carefully and individually planned for you. Any changes could drastically extend the completion of your program.

Appointments: — Take someone: On days with appointments to be seen by your doctor, you really should try to have a spouse or friend accompany you, for the doctor may give you several oral instructions that could be hard to remember.

Appointments: — Your questions: It is wise to jot down your questions as they arise. Be careful to write them fully enough for you to decipher when you are with the doctor. This is not the time for you to practice your shorthand or use just key words; sometimes abbreviations aren't enough to commit all of them to memory. Oh, and don't leave your list at home!

Centimeters vs. inches: It is easy to confuse centimeters and inches. One centimeter is about 3/8 of an inch, thus 2 centimeters about 3/4 of an inch and 5 centimeters is nearly 2 inches. The medical profession generally prefers to use international measurements for worldwide understanding, so don't get confused thinking your tumor is larger than it actually is.

Concern for family members: Many cancer centers have a geneticist on staff for those patients who are particularly concerned about their family members developing cancer. DNA testing now can be done to indicate risk levels.

Focus of doctors & nurses: Nurses and doctors are extremely busy yet most seem especially focused on every single patient they treat. Their recognition of this dedication to the care of everyone as an individual, rather than just another case, makes treatment days much more bearable.

Focus of patients & doctors: If patients and their physicians focus totally on cancer and its symptoms and treatments, never seeing each other as individuals, the disease may become a wall which separates rather than unites them. Each is left alone and wanting when the human connection is missing. Even a little TLC goes a long way. As with any authoritative figure, doctors must distance themselves somewhat from their patients in order to protect their own empathetic feelings. Fortunately most doctor-patient relationships find a successful middle ground.

Follow instructions: Prior to any surgery, you will be given oral and written instructions. You must follow them to the letter.

Girl Scouts quote:
Girl Scouts sing a song:

Make new friends but keep the old;
Some are silver and the others gold.

You will make new friends during your cancer treatments. They will help strengthen your determination to do whatever you must in order to become well again. Also, old friends from the past will surprise you with E-mails, telephone calls, cards, and prayers. Renewing old friendships is a thrill. Whoever would have thought that getting cancer could bring such unexpected blessings!

Grapefruit: Some health magazines have advised that certain drugs can cause serious problems in combination with grapefruit. A few varieties of sour oranges, such as Sevilles, seem to have an effect similar to that of grapefruit juice. It has been noted that substances in this fruit could cause a higher than prescribed amount of certain drugs to circulate through your bloodstream, which might possibly cause adverse reactions. It seems that a single eight ounce glass of grapefruit juice could cause an increased drug level in the blood, which remains in your body for three or more days. Most other citrus products are thought to be perfectly safe. Just be on guard about them and either abstain from their use or ask advice from your pharmacist or physician.

Interest or hobby: In your "best" days, you will be much happier if you already have a hobby or have developed a new interest to occupy your body and mind in restful ways. Tennis or other strenuous exercises may be out of the question for a while; however, reading is a given. Checking catalogs to shop ahead for Christmas and birthday gifts, knitting, writing, or painting, may be among things that you could pick up or set aside at any time. Such activities will stimulate your zest for life more than mindlessly watching television for hours.

Knowledge: Learn medical terminology at every opportunity. Understanding what chemicals are working for you and why they are being given will make taking them more meaningful. The reasoning behind the strong poisons it takes to kill cancer cells will allow you to realize the importance of going through the entire regimen. See Chapter 14 for a listing of some medical terms.

Love & support: More people love you than are able to show you their deep feelings; even more seem to be unable to put into words what you mean to them.

Mammogram — Digital: Digital mammography is a fairly new technology that allows images to appear instantly, reducing the need for some diagnostic biopsies. The hopes for the future start with the improvements of today.

Mammogram — Self-exam: Yearly mammograms certainly matter, but regular self-examinations are also extremely important. Whether you are a younger or older woman, select a particular day each month to be good to yourself by checking your breasts. If you are pre-menopausal, choose a date after your period. Perhaps your birth date or another meaningful day will jog your memory.

Metastatic breast cancer: If your breast cancer spreads to other parts of your body, it is still diagnosed by its original classification. Its appearance elsewhere would then be called metastatic breast cancer; even if it is found to have moved into your bones, it continues to be called breast cancer, not bone cancer. This definition also fits *local failure*, which means that cancer has appeared in the same breast.

Nicotine: If you smoke, be aware that nicotine constricts the blood vessels in your eyes as well as throughout your entire body. Your regular ingestion of vitamins A, C, and E can perform as your ACE safeguard in helping to protect your eyesight. Of course, not smoking is the smartest prevention of all.

No recovery: Those who will never completely recover from their types of cancer need recurring treatment to minimize their pain and prolong their quality of life. In this age, however, most cancer patients detect their tumors early enough that they can expect to be on the route to recovery.

Numbness: Most people who have had lymph nodes removed find that there is some numbness affecting the muscles of the upper arm and possibly the shoulder and back. Very gradually your body will regain some sensations, but entire normal feelings may take years or may never totally return. Exercising may help somewhat.

Offers of help: It is important to add here that some offers to help are merely polite acknowledgements of your condition of dependency from people who secretly hope that you won't ask anything of them. You'll probably suspect that this is true when they speak, and you might lightly say, "Be careful what you offer; next time I might ask something big of you." Then next time the ball will be in their court to offer help only if they are serious.

Pain patches or medications: Sometimes pain patches or medications can alter behavior drastically. Even if the prescribed portion is the normal dosage for most people, it can turn out to be too strong for your system. Occasionally a person may have reactions which cause her to respond to some medications exactly opposite from the prescribed manner anticipated. Let someone know at once if you experience this paradox or have any erratic thoughts or strange feelings such as disorientation, severe headaches, or vomiting. Notify your doctor so your situation can be appraised and your dosage can perhaps be altered.

Pesticides: With regard to pesticides on produce, of course it is always wise to wash all of your fresh vegetables and fruit before eating them. Although these items sometimes contain low levels of pesticides, the overall health benefits and cancer-protective effects of eating these treated items outweigh the risks involved. It may seem strange, but many people who were enthusiastic about fruit all their lives and less than thrilled with vegetables, have now found veggies to be wonderful, too. We can only hope that this love affair will continue for the rest of their lives, probably making them live even longer.

Platelets: Platelets are cells that create a clot to arrest bleeding at the site of an injury. People with low platelet counts are said to have thrombocytopenia. Physicians always check for this and, if found, treat it at once. Should you have any unusual bleeding or bruising, be sure to mention it promptly.

Prayer lists: Allow your name to be added to as many prayer lists as possible. It is widely believed that the power of prayer can indeed improve one's health.

Quiet day: Most people learn to enjoy a quiet day with nothing to do. Especially is this true if that "nothing" includes *not* having to leave home to receive a shot or treatment!

Radiation sickness: Constant over-exposure to x-rays and other radioactive material is dangerous and can cause radiation sickness. This is the reason that precision is so important with your treatments and also why all radiation teams must protect themselves by leaving the room each time you are treated. While they are nearby and busy monitoring you with their radiation equipment, they still can continuously see and hear you.

Research study: Young women with breast cancer are sometimes asked to join clinical trials. They may take part in research studies of new breast cancer treatments. Consider whether or not you would be willing to participate if your doctor suggests that you are an eligible candidate.

Responsible for your own health: No personal problems can be solved until individuals assume some responsibility for trying to help in finding a solution. This has to include one's own health care each day.

Risky medications: We all realize how expensive prescription medications are these days. It may be tempting but it is definitely risky to buy drugs from other countries or from any strangers. Perhaps pills procured online are accurately proportioned, but the chance of your being ripped off must be considered. Regardless of cost, your resulting good health is a bargain.

Say "Cancer": The very word *cancer* is frightening to everyone. It was a synonym for a death sentence years ago. Now medical science has progressed beyond that condemnation. The word itself is still shunned by many; but when the disease is yours, it must be acknowledged and used. The more often the word is spoken, the less power it has over you and your family.

Self-examinations: In self-examinations of your breasts, you should be searching for any hard mass that does not move around. Use smooth rotations of your flattened hand or the middle section of your index finger. Doing this frequently will more likely allow you to detect deviations from earlier inspections. If there is even a slight change, make an appointment with your physician.

Sex fears: Sexual experiences vary under ordinary circumstances and are likely to fluctuate during your illness due to both physical and emotional stress. Anxieties about health, family, finances, side effects, hormonal changes or a plethora of other problems can interfere with physical intimacy. You and your partner will continue to decide what is pleasurable and satisfying to you both at various times. Hugging and cuddling may be more important than ever, while more intimate activity may have to wait a while.

Sex problems: Cancer treatments often reduce the sexual desire in women. This is due to vaginal dryness which may make intercourse painful. Since some petroleum products may ccontribute to yeast infections, you may find safer vaginal lubricants near the feminine hygiene supplies. Now available are many water-based gels without irritating coloring or perfumes.

Shooting pain: Since cancer cells have no *brakes* of their own, as our growth cells do for height, they must be treated like weeds. They need to be removed from the body wherever they may show indications of sprouting. A shooting pain feels much like the swift headache that frozen drinks can cause when you swallow them too fast. If you feel that type of sudden pain in your breast, don't ignore it just because it lasts for only a few moments. Though uncommon, it may be a signal of trouble. Make a quick self-examination and an appointment with your oncologist for an immediate check-up.

Suggested gifts: Making a gift basket of small articles for your friends who are undergoing breast cancer treatments will be doubly welcomed. It will show your concern for them and start them off with items that you have found especially comforting. You may know what to give, but below are a few ideas you might consider.

Aloe cream	Altoids
Ballpoint pen	Bandana
Blank stickers	Boost (vanilla)
Chewing gum	Cornstarch
Daily journal	Dial soap

Gatorade	Handkerchiefs
Hard candy	Instant oatmeal
Jello	Magazines
Movies	Notepaper
Packages of ginger tea	Paperback books
Potted aloe plant	Pumice stone
Shower chair	Soft toothbrush
Stamps	Videos & DVDs

Naturally you'll want to include an obvious choice, this book [grin], since it has been written especially for you and your caregivers.

Trust doctor: Be assured that your doctor will not prescribe any treatment unless the benefits are greater than any known risks.

Uncomfortable: Whatever is wrong with your body during treatment, at first you will naturally assume that it is yet another side effect. Any strange or uncomfortable reactions could be symptoms caused by problems unrelated to your regimen. Sometimes it is difficult to detect the origin of concerns, but your doctor can suggest or prescribe remedies.

Vitamins, minerals, etc.: As of now, there is no scientific evidence that extra vitamins, minerals, or other dietary supplements will help fight cancer or stop it from recurring. If you ever consider taking an over-the-counter drug or anything other than that endorsed by your oncologist, check first for his or her opinion. Some vitamins may counteract the drugs being given during your regular treatment. Never

ever take any drug prescribed for someone else. Even if it is the same drug that your doctor has ordered for you, the other patient's dosage could be out-of-date, ineffective, and either stronger or weaker than your condition requires.

Weight gain: Although many cancer patients tend to lose weight, the treatments cause the opposite effect for some who may instead gain many pounds. If you are one who puts on weight during your treatment phase, know that during this time becoming healthy is more important than dieting or worrying about surplus pounds. Get well first and then concern yourself with gradually regaining your preferred weight, just as those who are too frail must also do.

Wheelchairs: During therapy some folks get so weak from fatigue or certain chemical mixtures that they require a wheelchair for a short time. Although this is rare, it is important to realize that it is almost always a temporary condition during their weakest moments. When your energy level rises, you will once again walk with normal endurance and agility.

White blood cells (WBC): These cells fight the germs that make people feel terrible. When there are too few WBCs, the patient has a deficiency called neutropenia. Your oncologist will give you complete blood counts (CBC) frequently; when the need is indicated, you could require a series of daily shots of Neupogen in order to rebuild these vital cells.

X-Rays vs. mammograms: The difference between mammograms and other x-rays is that mammograms show interior *tissue* while x-rays generally show *bone structure.* Ultrasound is another type of examination used to focus more closely on a specific area.

Your chemobrain: As a breast cancer patient you may become temporarily more forgetful than usual, but you'll have a handy excuse called *chemobrain.* This condition overrides other euphemisms such as "a senior moment" or "just too busy." Whatever the terminology, there is one nice thing that memory loss allows. If you read a "Who Done It" one week, a short time later you may read it again since you probably will have forgotten who was proven to be the murderer. So smile! We all need to find humor in situations thrust upon us; if we can just remember to keep grinning, *chemobrain* can be tolerated!

Your "CLOX" test: Some oncologists have found a quick test for those who seem to have developed chemically-induced memory loss, dementia, or *chemobrain.* Called the CLOX Test, its results alert your oncologist if more attention may be required. Here is the simple procedure: you will be asked to draw the face of a clock with its numbers and its hands set for a certain time. Your drawing will be interpreted immediately by your oncologist. This check is as uncomplicated as the physical examination that your primary doctor may give for determining your coordination, namely the test that requires you rapidly to touch your index finger to your nose, alternating right and left hands.

Your hazy days: When medications for young or old are involved, our bodies often protect us by making us woozy. This includes our being forgetful about important dates or promises, foggy about names we know well, and even unclear about whether we took the very pills that made us so absent-minded. During these times some people may experience deep sleep, strange dreams, and perhaps even a misty-eyed sensitivity to minor irritations. Understanding these reactions permits us to shrug off such behavior with an embarrassing chuckle. Anesthesia and medications allow our bodies to heal with as little pain as possible. In other words, don't be too hard on yourself while you are being treated.

Chapter 11

Support

AMERICAN CANCER SOCIETY

Always free services: As far as I know, there is never a fee for any ACS service. Their financial survival is completely funded through donations, corporate and individual, raised through honorariums and memorial legacies. For example, Winn-Dixie donated the first million ($1,000,000) to initiate the ACS Hope Lodge in Gainesville, FL. Some Hope Lodges elsewhere have similar partners from philanthropic foundations. Currently there are 25 Hope Lodges in the United States and Puerto Rico which provide temporary homes to patients undergoing cancer treatments.

Best support group: Anyone who has no attentive spouse, adult child, sister, or devoted friend could gain much comfort by joining one of the cancer support groups. Naturally, patients with supportive partners are also welcomed. Contact your local ACS for a schedule of their uplifting and informative meetings. Sign up early in your treatment.

Looking Good, Feeling Better: This beauty enrichment program allows ACS women to demonstrate coping tips that have been designed specifically for people going through chemotherapy or radiation treatments. "Look Good, Feel Better" includes appearance enhancement using cosmetics, wigs, scarves and turbans. Trained personnel give many free cosmetics to each participant as she is shown how to use these gifts in creative and skillful ways.

Reach for Recovery: Breast cancer survivors who have adjusted to their own diagnoses and treatments have volunteered to help you through this ACS program called "Reach For Recovery." These teachers are trained individuals, each of whom is matched with one patient at a time when you are facing emotional and physical challenges. You may request a visit at any time from your diagnosis and on through your recovery, breast reconstruction, and any recurrent cancer.

Relay charity walk: As one of many ACS programs, "Relay For Life" includes a charity walk as a blended celebration of cancer survivorship plus a fund raiser. It is held worldwide on dates set by individual chapters. This overnight event has the atmosphere of an altruistic party and a community spirit of unification for an important cause. It is a great mutual endeavor to join others while donating time, energy, and financial support for research and education. An added bonus is having a wonderful time together with both survivors and supporters.

Relay — Entire night: At Relay For Life events there is a carnival-like mood. There may be live music, balloons and other festive items, candy and special food for sale by various clubs, businesses, schools, churches, families and friends. Many people from these same groups form walking teams that have raised countless amounts of money through pledges and personal donations. ACS furnishes free printed tee-shirts for survivors and offers other shirts to the financial support teams to wear during their walks. Teams walk together or in shifts, while some individuals and groups walk all through the night. Most survivors and interested supporters stay as long as they are able. The track is never empty during the entire night and a hearty breakfast awaits the unfaltering dawn greeters. Tracks vary in length and types, depending upon the different parts of the country that participate. Traditionally, some of the 460,000 cancer survivors everywhere walk the first lap to start the relay. Most are on foot; but others appear with canes, walkers, or even wheelchairs.

Relay — I Can Cope: This ACS program is a combination lecture and discussion series of classes including topics on coping with problems facing the needs of people undergoing cancer. Your family members are encouraged to attend. Embraced are topics such as money matters, expressing feelings and fears, living within limitations, relieving both mental and physical pains, plus names of local resources. You will meet with other patients and share experiences which will become another support group for you.

Relay — Participate: There is shared enthusiasm when "Relay For Life" walkers applaud the survivors as they pass by them. The spectators and survivors thank all walkers in like manner. It is exciting to be among the participants and a pleasant surprise to find that many doctors, nurses, other staff members and their families join in these walks. Officially patients are designated as survivors if they have remained cancer free for five years after treatment is completed, but you will feel like a survivor each time you have a follow-up visit that shows no cancer has returned. You'll be thrilled when "Relay For Life" comes to your community. Look forward to it and promise yourself that you will participate!

Relay — Road to Recovery: Some ACS centers offer trained volunteer drivers to assist patients in need of rides to or from treatments. Check to see if this program entitled "Road To Recovery" might be a service given in your community. If you need transportation help, don't hesitate to call your local ACS to see if it is available.

Two more programs: "Tell A Friend" and "College & Camp Scholarships" are two other programs under the ACS sponsorship to be remembered. The first encourages their friends to get mammograms; the second provides tuition assistance to childhood cancer survivors. All ACS programs are underwritten by private and organizational donations.

CALL BY NAME
Nothing makes patients know that you care about them more than when you call them by name. Actually, whether we are healthy or not, we like that personal recognition.

CALLS TO DOCTOR
Non-professional caregivers or family members have one responsibility above all else. They are the ones who must contact the doctor if they feel you are in urgent need. Often caregivers ask the patient if the doctor should be called; frankly, patients usually are in no condition to make objective decisions. When family or friends are your health care providers and become worried or have doubts about your care, *they* should make the call rather than expecting you to be able to evaluate yourself.

CARDS

As simple as a greeting card or note may seem to the sender, it can brighten the entire day for the recipient.

CAREGIVERS

Be nice to them: Be extra nice to your caregivers and children. Everyone is under a great strain because they don't understand what you are going through and are unable to make you well with a magic wand. They feel thwarted when they can't do enough to ease your pain and that might cause them to become somewhat short-tempered.

Bless them: Bless all caregivers! It would be hard to cope without them. Whether they are your mate, parents, adult children or other relatives, friends or paid helpers, they are all saints in thinly-veiled disguises.

Express feelings: Attention, caregivers: especially during those dreaded five days right after chemotherapy, patients need tangible expressions of love and other caring signs.

Thank often: Caregivers are only temporary helpers to your every request because they love you and wish they could take away your pain. Try to remember to say your P's and Q's (Please and Thank Q's). Without those words, requests tend to sound more like orders and aren't as well received.

CHORES

When loved ones ask if they can help you, know that they really do want a suggestion. Try to think of small chores such as taking care of a load of laundry, changing the water in flower vases, clipping a hedge that blocks a view or otherwise annoys you, or making a needed telephone call for you. Even pulling your curtains opened or closed, or bringing you a glass of fresh water will suffice. Little things help them feel less frustrated and more needed.

DOCTORS

There are times when physicians must be somewhat aloof with patients due to pressures of time and empathy for your condition. They sometimes must conceal their innermost feelings of compassion and helplessness, especially with chronically ill people, in order to continue treating them with dignity. God bless both the doctors and the patients.

FLOWERS

Don't handle yet: Should you handle live flowers during the early days of treatment? This is a "no-no" because their fragrance can make you feel queasy and their prickly leaves or thorns can cause infections. Just let your caregiver and friends tend to them for now. Enjoy flowers from a distance and let others arrange your bouquets for you. That is one of the nice things you can delegate to others which will let them know that they are needed and appreciated.

Morale: Farther along in your treatment, you may enjoy fresh cut flowers. When you are feeling much better and run out of flowers, there are no rules posted anywhere saying that you can't buy some for yourself to boost your own morale.

FRIENDSHIPS

Bless them all: Everyone is so very busy these days, but some of your best support will come when friends and family telephone, E-mail, send cards, or visit in person. Every single time that someone takes a moment to do anything personal for you, it lightens your spirits and makes you know that they haven't forgotten you and that they are praying for your recovery in a special way. God bless them all!

Develop them: Unexpected friendships sometimes develop with unexplained ease under unforeseen circumstances.

Empathy: Sometimes people really do need friends and family to empathize with them in their pain and suffering. They may not admit it because most of the time patients prefer to be uplifting and uplifted; however, if they are really depressed, sincere empathy will be accepted as understanding. Cleansing tears may flow from them and even from you, and that's okay. Never ever forget the power of hugs! They transmit your emotions at comforting times as well as during joyful ones.

GROUPS

There are many avenues to explore if you feel the desire for a support group. Your local Cancer Society, a hospital chaplain, or even an internet support group may be the right one for you. One thing to remember is that some groups will not suit you, but if you keep trying you are sure to find a perfect fit for your needs.

JOKES

Often forwarded E-mail jokes and pictures from family and friends really do help lighten the spirits of most patients, but personal notes and messages are welcomed even more heartily.

LONELINESS

Only loneliness in the extreme can kill the desire for humans to fight for their lives. We must let no one feel so lonely or forsaken.

PRAYERS QUOTE

Prayers are powerful. It is humbling yet a grand feeling to know that people are raising your name in prayer to a loving God. You can also pray for Him to stay near you through these difficult times. Believe that there are more things brought about by prayer than you can imagine and you will not be surprised when they are forthcoming. In Matthew 7:7 we have been promised, *Ask and it shall be given unto you.*

SHARING

Sharing different cancer experiences and tested techniques may help patients consider alternatives for themselves.

SUPPORTIVE WORDS

If you really want to encourage a breast cancer patient, tell her how very brave she is and how inspiring her strength is to her friends and family. The law of expectation will make her cope even better. It works with children who are praised when they do things we are proud of and it will make her just as eager to continue to be appreciated for her courage.

VISITS

Do keep short: After surgery and subsequent treatments, have your family suggest a limit of 15 minutes or less for bedside visitors. You don't need to be entertaining during those first down days. Concentrate on resting and healing yourself. Later, when friends want to visit, suggest that they call first to be sure you are feeling well enough to enjoy the time you plan to spend together. Don't be afraid to say that a later date might be better if you are feeling too ill to welcome their visit on a "bad" day.

How to keep short: When friends come to visit and stay too long, simply tell them that it's time for your nap. They will understand. If they still don't leave or you don't feel comfortable saying anything, just slide down a bit, close your eyes, and doze off to sleep. They'll get that message soon enough and not even think you are rude.

VULNERABILITY

You will make friends with many other people during your treatments. Some will be fatally ill and may even need to have Hospice care. It is very difficult to lose friends to death and doubly hard when you have watched their gallant fight to survive. Further, their demise is a sharp reminder that you also are in a vulnerable state. The best thing you can do for fatally ill friends is to comfort their families. Your being their support will strengthen your resolve to do all you can to become a survivor for your own family.

Chapter 12

Attitude

"BAD, BETTER, BEST" DAYS

If you are taking chemotherapy for the 21-day cycle, try this:

+ Call your physically hardest first five days after chemotherapy your "bad" days.
+ After those "bad" days have passed, call the next five "better" days.
+ Then call the next ten or eleven days "best" days. This probably will help put things in perspective, giving you some assurance and consolation that the "better" to "best" stages far outnumber the others.

If your treatment schedule differs from the cycle mentioned above, you will find your own pattern of "bad, better, best" days. You then can identify and anticipate your upcoming "better" and "best" days.

CHEERFULNESS

A cheerful attitude goes a long way toward your feeling better, even if you have to fake it sometimes. It helps both you and all others to acknowledge that you are fighting for better health because life is good. Your expressions of good spirits are contagious and allow relatives and friends to be less stressed over your cancer.

CHOICES

Free will: Oncologists do their part in ridding your body of cancer. Our own free will allows us to make a conscious effort regarding trouble; that is, not to borrow trouble by worrying about things we can neither predict nor change. A much more positive approach is to accept your present condition and be grateful for treatments available to help us resume better health. An uplifting attitude won't cure you, but it will go a long way in keeping you eager to beat this disease.

Ultimately: Each of us must live with the choices we make in all aspects of life - especially regarding our positive and negative attitudes, which ultimately are also our own choices.

COURAGE

First Days: Usually the first few days after chemotherapy require much courage. They are equivalent to super flu plus morning sickness for women and super flu plus kidney stones for men. Once those miserable days pass, things get more bearable. That's a promise!

Surprise: You'll find more courage living in your soul than you ever imagined you possessed. What a wonderful deep-seated surprise!

EXPRESSION

Someone has said, "Of all the things we wear, our facial expressions are the most important." Surely you'll agree.

FEARS

Family members must allow patients to talk openly about their alarming fears. There are different fears with different phases of treatment. After your diagnosis, you probably felt shock and anger, disbelief, or numbing amazement. During your treatment undoubtedly you will worry over your chronic fatigue and all the other possible side effects. You may also be upset if you encounter any unexpected bodily disfigurement. You will be especially anxious about your unjustified guilt trips in regard to your spouse and the possibility of genes carrying cancer to your descendants. Anticipating these fears allows you to face them one at a time.

FRIENDS

Bonding: The ability of the soul to include more friends into your list of people for whom you care will certainly expand. Must we become dreadfully ill before we truly realize how special all the people are who share our earth and our lives? No!

Busy: Remember how busy your healthy friends are. Do not feel hurt if you don't see them as often as you had expected. They haven't forgotten you, but are probably as involved with their own lives as you recently were with yours. Try to understand and not make them feel guilty. We all do the best we can.

HAIR

When you have no hair, it is surprising how much you notice the lovely sheen and hair styles of healthy people. You automatically begin looking to the future and wondering what fashion will look best when you regain your own hair.

HELP OTHERS

Cancer promotes introspection, allowing us meditation time which leads us to see others with a more caring heart. There are many frightened people looking eagerly for a friendly face who will recognize their needs and respond to them. Cancer and other diseases instill a deeper desire to reach out and make a difference by helping others.

HUGS

People love the human touch. Hugs are wonderful but a pat on the back is mighty good, too.

IMAGINATION

Be an informed patient. Imagination is much more fearful than any facts you'll learn.

LIMITS

Know your limitations during treatment and recovery stages. You are not being lazy when you are unable to do things that formerly seemed effortless. With the passing of time and self-care, you will gradually adapt as your energy strengthens.

LISTEN

Reach out with a sympathetic ear to other patients with understanding and an encouraging attitude. New cancer patients need to talk with more seasoned patients.

MACHINES

Sometimes treatment machinery breaks down with a glitch that requires adjustments, just like any computer does. Then highly specialized mechanics are called to make repairs. Delays are essential to assure precision maintenance. Patience is required of all. Just recognize the fact that not only you but also the medical staff will be expected to remain later than they had planned.

MEMORY

When memory fails and your brain cells seem blank and uncooperative, try to be forgiving of yourself most of all. Understand that you are in the midst of learning a lesson in cancer management. Everything will improve once you complete this tough educational course.

MIRRORS

Mirrors are not to be avoided. Face reality. Look directly into your mirror and make your eyes sparkle with life because your *ill* days are *killing* the evil cancer cells.

OTHERS

As ill as you might feel on any given day, when you go for your treatment you may find other patients who are much sicker than you are. That probably will result in your reviewing your own plight with thanksgiving and offering up prayers for those who are worse off than you. It's amazing how we prefer to face our own most difficult challenges rather than trade places with someone else.

PAIN

Current events: Keep up with current events and you'll find yourself thinking more often of everyday happenings. You'll put your friends at ease if your conversation dwells on subjects other than your aches and pains. Talk instead with them about their lives and activities. This will make for happier times together.

Groaning: Try hard not to *be* a pain when you have pains. Your family members will appreciate it, even though they understand that you are aching and frustrated. If you find some comfort in groaning softly, however, that is allowed. Just don't overdo it!

PATIENCE

Frankly, each of us must remember that when we don't feel well, we tend to become short on patience and rather irritable. Admit this to yourself and try to curb your irrational behavior when unexpected impulses occur.

PLAN

Planning your "after treatment vacation" is an up-beat way to spend your rest periods. Even listing short-term hopes, such as renting a certain video or driving to a park, can project your imagination into a feasible goal. Short day trips on your "best" days can make you feel part of the mainstream of life.

PMS

Occasionally your spirits will wilt and need boosting. Expect to find yourself very suddenly irritated or weepy over trivialities. Taking a nap will help you regain control over these mood changes. This particular type of PMS can hit men as well as women. If you rename it for the men, just call it Personal Misery Syndrome.

POWER

Knowledge is power that will allow you to feel more in control. Learn all that you can about cancer treatments and ways that can help you cope with the temporary changes in your life.

PRAY CASSETTES

Cassettes: If you are unable to attend your church, you may consider asking the secretary if sermon cassettes are available, or find a Sunday message being shown on television or broadcast on the radio.

Doctors: Doctors are humans who tend to our needs, share our joys, grieve with us and those we love, and they desperately want us to regain vital health. Let's remember them in our nightly prayers.

PRIORITIES TOP BILLING

In case people didn't have their priorities in order before they were diagnosed, they soon learn to rearrange them. Golf, bridge, or whatever earlier seemed so important all become trivial and fall way down on the list. Top billing goes to good health as well as to a deeper appreciation of and closer relationships with family and friends. Patients especially will develop an amazing personal pride in strengths that they never realized they possessed.

REJOICE

Rejoice in the thought that your responsibility to your body's well-bring depends on *you*. A strong faith, nourishment with food supplements when needed, enormous amounts of liquids (especially water, no alcohol), much rest between cancer treatments, plus a positive attitude will soon allow you to feel a lot better. It is ultimately your determination that will lead you to follow the required path back to a healthy future. Vow not to give up along the way.

SAY IT

Don't talk in euphemisms such as "this dreaded disease," "my condition," or "my troubles." Its power over you lessens when you call it the evil thing that it is! Say the hated word, *cancer*.

SCARS FADING

Thankfully, there are numerous creams and prescription treatments available that will help hide scars. It will amaze you how quickly your surgical scars fade. Our bodies have miraculous restorative powers. Remembering this throughout the treatments will reinforce your positive faith in both body and attitude.

SELF-PITY TEARS

Some tunes may remind you of your younger days when you were healthier and more carefree. Self-pity invites tears. Sometimes a good cry is to be expected. Just promise yourself not to linger too long in the "poor me" stage.

SKETCH

Imagine a sketched figure of yourself being "normal" again and visualize your current self stepping into that outlined being. That is a goal to anticipate and to expect after the cancer is vanquished.

STRENGTH VICARIOUS

When you see golfers, tennis players, or joggers, try to enjoy their energy vicariously and promise yourself that you will be that strong again soon. Meanwhile, be certain not to run anywhere as your balance may be a bit off center.

TERMS

Learning medical terms will help you understand your condition and make you feel more in control of your situation, especially if you add your individual medications to the list of terms mentioned herein. Feel free to ask your doctor or clinical nurse about the purposes and possible side effects of all your drugs. You'll find everyone on the staff to be very cooperative.

THANKS

Thank your spouse, partner, parents, children, and friends often for all the help and love that they give to you so freely. This tells them that you care about them and appreciate their continuing support.

TWINKLING EYES

Just take a look in your mirror, then think of something especially pleasant; your eyes will light up and your entire expression will become more appealing. You'll find that other people are magnetically attracted to you when your eyes twinkle. Allow your natural enthusiasm for life to shine forth while compelling gloomy thoughts to cease. Show your sparkle, thereby helping those who love you to deal more easily with your cancer as they sense how well you are coping.

WAIT

When you must wait to be seen at the medical center, be aware that especially sick men, women, and children sometimes require more time than was anticipated. Try to be tolerant and understanding. Attempt to put yourself in the shoes of those patients who need extra time that day.

WEAKNESS

A good attitude is important, but feeling weak or faint is another story altogether. Don't feel you are babying yourself if you need to lie down while waiting for your treatment. Tell a nurse. There may be a cot or recliner available.

Chapter 13

Sources of Interest

AMERICAN CANCER SOCIETY

Close by: Almost every town in the country has a branch of the ACS. They have many varied programs and support groups for cancer patients and caregivers. Check your local telephone directory or ask your physician.

Free: If you visit the ACS you'll be offered some caps and wigs – free! Wearing them will protect your baldness from the weather while allowing a good variety for you. Your selections may later be returned, passed on to other people, or kept for yourself.

ANGEL FLIGHT NETWORK

Corporate Angel Network, Inc. is a nationwide public charity which serves economically needy people. You should know about it if you must be treated at a cancer center far from your residence, for you might otherwise find the cost of commercial air travel to be financially prohibitive. The Angel Network may be able to arrange passage for cancer patients to distant treatment centers by using empty seats offered by some businesses on their corporate jets. Prospective patients may wish to communicate with this volunteer service by calling toll free 1-800-352-4256 or for corporate jet service at number 1-866-328-1313. Instead of phoning, if you have a computer contact them online at <u>www.corpangelnetwork.org/</u>

CANCER SURVIVORS' NETWORK

The Cancer Survivors' Network exists for you. It promises anonymity and accessibility to survivors and their families, caregivers, and all whose lives have been affected emotionally through this disease. Survivors who are willing to share their experiences are readily available to help you cope with this challenge. Their services include radio talk shows with conversations and interviews, personal stories, and hope for today and the future. Comfort may be right at your finger tips by going online to <u>www.cancer.org</u> or by phone at 1-877-333-4673.

HOPE LODGES

Accommodations: If your treatments require you to move temporarily to another town, try to determine if a Hope Lodge may be located there. They are sponsored by the American Cancer Society plus certain commercial and/or institutional organizations for cancer patients but *only* while they are receiving treatment.

Buy your own food: Each patient undergoing treatment plus one companion will have the use of private living quarters. All that you will be required to do is buy your own food and follow the house rules. The concern of daily living becomes one less worry for you. The companionship of fellow residents will lift your spirits as you develop friendships with other patients and caregivers who understand well what you are feeling and experiencing.

Finances: Everything is offered totally free; however, if you are financially able to give donations at any time, they will be gratefully accepted. Such contributions will forever perpetuate this magnanimous service to even more patients. For questions regarding free housing during cancer treatments, telephone 1-800-ACS-2345 or use the Internet at www.cancer.org.

Similar facilities: If there is no Hope Lodge in your area, check to see if there is a similar accommodation. Several large cancer centers or hospitals may have available residence facilities nearby.

HOSPICE

Purpose: When you or someone you care about is facing death, be sure to ask a doctor about a Hospice organization nearest you. It provides sensitive palliative care for people with advanced diseases. Call toll free to 1-800-299-4677, use your computer at www.hospicemsl.org or contact their E-mail at info@hospicemsl.org.

Services: These services rendered by Hospice organizations all across America include the following wonderful care, regardless of your ability to pay:

+Adult day respite
+Availability 24 hours a day 7 days a week
+Final residential care in many areas
+Free grief counseling
+Home health aides
+Pain management
+Pharmacy services
+Physician home visits
+Spiritual & emotional care

LIFE IS GOOD

Cling to hope and never give up. The good of living is too precious to abandon freely. Incidentally, there is a neat T-shirt company called *Life Is Good* at www.lifeisgood.com. Each comical drawing on their various colored shirts reminds us of the truth of their company name.

NATIONAL CANCER INSTITUTE (NCI) : FINANCIAL AID

If you need financial aid, contact a hospital social service office or NCI Cancer Information Service and telephone toll free to 1-800-4-CANCER (1-800-422-6237.) They may be able to help pay for some of your treatments or possibly direct you to other sources of help. Visit your local social services office regarding the Medicaid program to discover if you are eligible.

NATIONAL LYMPHEDEMA NETWORK

Information about lymphedema will be found by clicking onto their web page at www.lymphnet. org/or by calling the National Lymphedema Network at 1-800 541-3259.

Chapter 14

Medical Terms

Advance Directive
Alkylamines
Anorexia
Aspirate
Autoimmune Disorder
Axillary
Benign
Biopsy
Brachytherapy
Breast-Conserving Surgery
Cancer
Carcinoma
Chemotherapy
Clinical Trial
Complete Blood Count (CBC)
CT "CAT" Scan

Cyst
Deoxyribonucleic Acid (DNA)
Digital Mammography
Ducts
Ductal Carcinoma In Situ
Early Therapy
Edema
Estrogen
Femara & Arimidex (Generic: Letrozole & Anastrozole)
Fibromyalgia
Fine-Needle Aspiration or Needle Biopsy
Follow-up Care
Gamma-Delta T Cells
Gynecologist
Hormonal Therapy
Hormonal Replacement Therapy (HRT)
Hormones
Hospice
Hydrocortisone
Inflammatory Breast Cancer
Intravenous Line (IV)
Invasive or Infiltrating Cancer
Lactose
Lobe
Lobular Carcinoma In Situ (LCIS)
Lumpectomy
Lupus
Lymph Nodes

Lymphedema
Magnetic Resonance Imaging (MRI)
Malignant
Mammogram
MammoSite
Mastectomy
Metastasis
Modified Radical Mastectomy
Neupogen (Generic: Filgrastim)
Oncology
Oncology Specialists
Paget's Disease
Pathologist
Petechiae
Physical Therapist
Physician's Assistant (PA)
Platelets
Port or Portal (Port-A-Cath)
Procrit (Generic: Epoetin Alpha)
Radiation
Radical or Halsted Radical Mastectomy
Radiologist
Recurrent Cancer
Sentinel Lymph Nodes
Sentinel Lymph Nodes Biopsy
Shunt
Stages of Breast Cancer
Tamoxifen
Thrombocytopenia

Tumor
Ultrasound
White Blood Cell (WBC)
White Blood Count
X-Ray

ADVANCE DIRECTIVE

A written or oral notice stating whether or not you want to receive any treatment is required by you or your designated appointee. This form also names the people whom you want to make treatment decisions in the event that you become unable to speak for yourself.

ALKYLAMINES

These "gamma-delta T cells," made in the bone marrow, aid the immune system by fighting bacteria and invasive germs.

ANOREXIA

A loss of appetite over a prolonged period that can become a life-threatening disease.

ASPIRATE

The withdrawing of fluids from a nipple, cyst, lump or other area where bodily fluids have accumulated.

AUTOIMMUNE DISORDER

A condition in which a misdirected immune system fights the body's own tissues.

AXILLARY

Pertaining to the area under the arm, including lymph nodes.

BENIGN

Non-cancerous.

BIOPSY

Procedure to remove cells or tissues for signs of disease.

BRACHYTHERAPY

A method whereby internal radiation is localized to the tumor site.

BREAST-CONSERVING SURGERY

Lumpectomy: removal of a tumor only.

Quadrantectomy: removal of one quarter of a breast.

Segmental mastectomy: removal of the cancer plus some breast tissue around the tumor and the lining of the chest muscles below the tumor.

CANCER

A disease in which abnormal cells divide and spread uncontrollably. Cancer cells can invade nearby tissues and spread throughout the bloodstream and lymphatic system.

CARCINOMA

Cancer that begins in the skin or in tissues lining or covering internal organs.

CHEMOTHERAPY

The medically supervised treatment with chemical drugs used to kill cancer cells.

CLINICAL TRIAL

A research study to test how well new medical treatments react.

COMPLETE BLOOD COUNT (CBC)

A simple test for checking blood cells.

CT (CAT) SCAN

A computer-generated cross-section view of a patient's anatomy.

CYST

A fluid-filled sac which, after aspiration and a check of the fluid, may be examined to determine if cells are benign or malignant.

DEOXYRIBONUCLEIC ACID (DNA)

One of two molecules that encode genetic information within the body of each individual and make you *you*.

DIGITAL MAMMOGRAPHY

A current method of rapid imaging which lessens the need for some biopsies.

DUCTS

Tubes through which body fluids pass.

DUCTAL CARCINOMA IN SITU

Abnormal cells that involve only the lining of a duct.

EARLY THERAPY

Treatment given before surgery to shrink tumors.

EDEMA

Swelling of soft tissues as a result of excess fluid accumulation.

ESTROGEN
A female hormone.

FEMARA & ARIMIDEX (Generic: Letrozole & Anastrozole)
Two hormone drugs that inhibit the production of estrogen.

FIBROMYALGIA
A syndrome that causes extreme fatigue and chronic pain without detectable inflammation.

FINE-NEEDLE ASPIRATION OR NEEDLE BIOPSY
Removal by needle of tissue or fluid for examination.

FOLLOW-UP CARE
Regular checkups which ensure that any changes in health are noticed by your doctor.

"GAMMA-DELTA T" CELLS
White blood cells that are cancer-fighting Alkylamines.

GYNECOLOGIST
A medical doctor who specializes in the treatment of women.

HORMONAL THERAPY

Treatment of cancer by removing, blocking, or adding hormones.

HORMONE REPLACEMENT THERAPY (HRT)

Hormones (estrogen and/or progesterone) given to post-menopausal women in order to replace the estrogen no longer produced by the ovaries. Those who have had their ovaries surgically removed are included in this group.

HORMONES

Chemicals produced by glands which circulate through the bloodstream and control action of certain cells and organs.

HOSPICE

An organization that provides expert and compassionate end-of-life care in many communities.

HYDROCORTISONE

A synthetic medication used as a replacement for adrenal insufficiency and in the treatment of various diseases associated with inflammation.

INFLAMMATORY BREAST CANCER

A disease in which the skin surface may look pitted. The breast becomes red, swollen, and warm to the touch due to the cancer cells blocking the lymph vessels in the skin.

INTRAVENOUS LINE (IV)

An access line into a vein for injecting drugs or drawing blood samples.

INVASIVE OR INFILTRATING CANCER

Any cancer that has spread beyond the layer of tissue in which it developed and is growing into surrounding healthy tissues.

LACTOSE

A sugar present in milk and other dairy products.

LOBE

Any portion of an organ such as the brain, breast, liver, lung, or even an ear.

LOBULAR CARCINOMA IN SITU (LCIS)

Abnormal cells found in the lobules of the breast. This condition seldom becomes invasive cancer; however, there is an increased risk of developing breast cancer in either breast.

LUMPECTOMY

Breast surgery to remove a tumor and some portion of the normal tissue surrounding it.

LUPUS

A chronic inflammatory disease caused by autoimmune conditions that allow antibodies in the blood to damage a person's own body tissues.

LYMPH NODES

Small bean-shaped organs located in the lymphatic system. They store special cells that can trap bacteria or cancer cells traveling through the body in lymph fluid. Clusters of these nodes are found in lymph glands in the underarms, groin, chest, neck, and abdomen.

LYMPHEDEMA

If lymph nodes are removed during surgery, this condition may develop causing your surgery arm and hand to become puffy and swollen. This happens when lymphatic fluid cannot drain properly. It is more likely to occur if you require radiation but can develop right after surgery, within a few months, or even years later.

MAGNETIC RESONANCE IMAGING (MRI)

A procedure in which a magnet linked to a computer is used to create detailed pictures of areas inside the body.

MALIGNANT

Cancerous.

MAMMOGRAM

An x-ray of the breast

MAMMOSITE

A radiation therapy system (RTS) that delivers radiation within the space left after a cancerous tumor is removed and also into the tissue directly surrounding that cavity where tumors are most likely to recur.

MASTECTOMY

Surgery to remove an entire breast.

METASTASIS

The spread of cancer from one part of the body to another.

MODIFIED RADICAL MASTECTOMY

Surgery to remove the entire breast, some of the lymph nodes under the arm, and the lining of the chest muscles. In some cases parts of the muscles in the chest wall are also removed.

NEUPOGEN (Generic: Filgrastim)
A drug sometimes injected to increase a patient's white blood count.

ONCOLOGY
The field of medicine that specializes in treating cancer with surgery, chemotherapy, radiation, and hormone therapy.

ONCOLOGY SPECIALISTS
Highly specialized doctors with advanced training in caring for cancer patients, plus their assistants: nurse practitioners, clinical nurses, or nurse specialists.

PAGET'S DISEASE
A form of breast cancer in which the tumor grows from ducts beneath the nipple onto the surface. Symptoms commonly include itching, burning and an eczema-like condition or even some oozing or bleeding around the nipple.

PATHOLOGIST
A doctor who identifies diseases by studying cells and tissues under a microscope.

PETECHIAE
The appearance of small spots on the skin of some patients which alert their doctors to a low platelet count.

PHYSICAL THERAPIST
A trained practitioner who is officially certified to administer individualized rehabilitative programs using equipment and exercises specifically designed for patients recovering their health.

PHYSICIAN'S ASSISTANT (PA)
One who provides medical care under the supervision of a physician.

PLATELETS
Cells that create a clot to arrest bleeding.

PORT OR PORTAL (PORT-A-CATH)
A surgically implanted access system whereby fluid medications go directly into a vein. In this manner, chemicals can be sent into your bloodstream through direct injections instead of using IVs.

PROCRIT (Generic: Epoetin Alpha)
A drug injected to build up diminishing red blood counts.

RADIATION

Delivery by external high-energy beams or implanted seeds to a specific area of the body in order to diagnose or shrink tumors and to kill cancer cells.

RADICAL OR HALSTED RADICAL MASTECTOMY

Surgery to remove the breast, chest muscles, and all lymph nodes under the arm. This operation is currently done only when the tumor has spread to the chest muscles.

RADIOLOGIST

Certified practitioner who uses x-rays, ultrasound, mammograms, and other imaging methods to locate, diagnose and treat diseases.

RECURRENT CANCER

The disease has returned.

SENTINEL LYMPH NODES

The first nodes that cancer is likely to invade as it spreads from the primary tumor.

SENTINEL LYMPH NODES BIOPSY

A procedure in which a dye or radioactive substance is injected near the tumor.

SHUNT

A temporary device that drains fluids from one part of the body to another.

STAGES OF BREAST CANCER

Determined by the extent of a cancer and whether or not it has metastasized.

TAMOXIFEN

An oral drug inhibiting estrogen from binding with cancer cell receptors.

THROMBOCYTOPENIA

A condition sometimes found in cancer patients with low platelet counts.

TUMOR

Any abnormal mass of tissue that results from excessive cell division. Tumors may be either benign or malignant.

ULTRASOUND

High frequency sound waves that are bounced off tissues allowing echoes to be converted into a picture.

WHITE BLOOD CELL (WBC)

A cell that fights body infections.

WHITE BLOOD COUNT
The actual count of white blood cells.

X-RAY
High energy radiation used in low doses to diagnose diseases and in high doses to treat cancer.

Chapter 15

Personal Anecdotes

A HALLOWEEN COSTUME

Hope was hairless when she received her final cancer treatment on Halloween. She chose to dress as an animal, her way of celebrating her graduation and bringing a smile to other patients. In costume, she asked that a friend paint brown and orange tiger stripes on her head to enhance the outfit. With makeshift ears, nose, and bushy oscillating tail, Hope demonstrated spunk and joy to many folks that day. One woman drew her aside to tell her that she too was ready to fight for recovery, inspired by a fighting tiger! Hope then disclosed the fact that her idea was spawned by a story she recalled.

It seems there are three things one can do when confronted by a wild tiger - a person can take flight, ignore, or fight the beast. Of course, if you take flight or ignore a tiger, you will likely lose; however, when you fight you have a chance of intimidating him and living longer.

People who have hope and fight to win their battles also have the greatest chance of living healthy lives. Hope's parents named her well!

A PAKISTANI DAUGHTER

Rubi, a recent graduate of medical school, was a young Pakistani living a normal happy life with her husband and child in Australia when she developed cancer of one eyelid. Sadly, no one in her part of the world was trained to treat her rare form of the disease. Eventually she learned about Shands Hospital and Hope Lodge in Florida. She was accepted immediately both as a patient by a team of oncologists and as a resident at that free temporary home. While living there she became friends with other patients, especially with Mary. Rubi cooked some of her special Pakistani meals for Mary and they also shared stories and pictures of their families. Four weeks of chemotherapy later, Rubi's oncologists regretfully agreed that she had come too late for effective treatment and suggested that she return to her family. Rubi responded only once to Mary's E-mails, saying, "Please pray for me." In vain, Mary prayed for Rubi and for further contact with her. As the months became years and her hopes of locating her friend dwindled, Mary recalled Rubi's warm embrace and farewell words, "You will always have a daughter in Australia." Now Mary fears that the ultimate conclusion must be that her Pakistani-Australian "daughter" can live only within her heart.

A SHARING OFFER

Helen suffered radiation side effects in the form of an itchy rash. Her doctor prescribed an ointment which helped considerably. Since her father Zach's aging skin was scaly from years of sun exposure, Helen suggested that he try her great moisturizing salve. He refused with a shrug. Zach seemed to feel that applying lubricants was not a masculine thing to do. Helen's comment was that he would have accepted it immediately if the medication had been a black or purple liniment that smelled to high heaven!

BIRTHDAY CAKE

When Casey's October birthday happened to fall on one of her chemotherapy days, she decided to treat her health care team with a special cake. The icing atop the cake depicted her zodiac sign *scorpion*, along with the Cancer zodiac symbol *crab*. Both scorpion and crab were drawn wearing boxing gloves and it was clear that the scorpion was getting the best of the crab. Casey's positive attitude was clearly revealed through her chosen theme. Her health team enjoyed exhibiting the unusual design to other patients before sharing slices of the symbolic cake with everyone present.

BUNNY

No joke! While his wife Phyllis, a chemo patient, was in the hospital with an infection at Easter, Jared brought her a candy-filled basket and some clip-on bunny ears. Her spirits were brightened and her sense of humor was renewed. She decided to add some fun into her bald life in a grand way. Donning her bunny ears, Phyllis walked from room to room accompanied by her IV pole, distributing candy to other patients on her floor. She looked purposely silly as she spread pleasure for the patients and staff. This altruistic mission also reminded everyone that in times of both joy and trouble God Incarnate is in our midst to help us cope with all of life's trials.

COUNTDOWN

Her oncologist told Anne that she would probably need a total of six treatments but, depending upon her progress, she might require two additional ones. Anne decided to devise a "Chemos To Go" countdown pad. She put eight pages together with Chemo # 8 on top and Chemo # 1 on the bottom. Her point was to tear off pages calendar-style after each procedure until the treatment days were all completed. Anne reasoned that if eight treatments were required, it wouldn't be such a mental letdown for her if she prepared eight pages to tear off. On the other hand, what a thrilling boost she would enjoy if the doctor decided that the final two possible treatments were unnecessary; then she could pull Chemo #3, Chemo #2, and Chemo #1 all at once!

EPIPHANY MOMENT

Cathy was lying prone in her bed suffering from unrelenting vomiting and nightly insomnia due to the side effects of her cancer treatments. She remembered from past treatments that, even though she was in her worst days, tomorrow would be better. She unconsciously flung her right hand into the air toward the ceiling, bringing to her mind Michelangelo's famous painting, *The Creation of Man*, in the Sistine Chapel. Instinctively, she began to pray, wishing that she too could touch the hand of God. In that moment, her index finger became hot! What an epiphany! God *is* ever-present. Silently weeping with amazement and joy, she realized that she was not alone, for God Himself had come to comfort her.

FUN WITH A RED WIG

For some years Amy dyed her hair red. When her mother became a cancer patient and sent a picture of herself wearing a red wig, the daughter responded, "It looks great! Now if anyone questions the natural color of *my* hair, I'll just show them a picture of my red-headed mom!"

GENES

Because Debbie had breast cancer, she planned to tell her oncologist about her concern over the possibility of her children getting it. Before she could phone him, her ever-inquisitive five-year old Malia asked, "Brother's eyes are green. Why are mine blue?" Mother Debbie explained, "You have your daddy's blue eyes but your brother got mommy's green genes." Minutes later Malia returned and wanted to know why they didn't all just wear blue jeans!

GOOD FRIENDS TAKE A LOT

One afternoon Jan and Hal dropped by to visit their good friends, Nan and Jeff. Nan was still undergoing regular chemotherapy and had lost all of her hair, but so far Hal had not seen her bald. On this particular day, Nan was wearing a cute black wig. Soon after they entered the living room, Jeff took Hal into another part of the house on some pretext. Nan proceeded to tell Jan of a cooked-up plan she and Jeff had concocted to tease Hal. Jan joined in the plotted scheme. As the men rejoined their wives, Jeff said, "Nan, that shortcut wig is especially attractive on you; don't you agree, Hal?" His response was, "Definitely nice." At that remark, his wife turned and said, "Well, let's see how it looks on me!" and yanked the wig from Nan's head, thereby revealing that bald head to poor Hal. He was aghast at his wife's behavior and surprised at Nan's changed appearance at the same time. He nearly fainted from shock until everyone else laughed so hard that they had to tell him it was a set-up.

IN MY SOUP

At one Hope Lodge, Awilde, a Puerto Rican woman, was distressed as her body began changing in reaction to her treatments. Her husband was coming the following day for a weekend visit and she wanted to look her best. Since time was of the essence, her friend Harriet gave Awilde one of her wigs, a blonde one, saying that she looked like Marilyn Monroe. Giggling, Awilde accepted the wig gratefully and hugged Harriet, saying, "Did you know that you are in all my soups?" Of course her friend figured that it was some sort of thank you, but Awilde clarified further. It's a Puerto Rican idiom referring to everyday soup served as a meal, meaning that Harriet will always be in her thoughts and heart! Cancer patients find unity in diversity and diversity in unity. We can learn and thrive from listening to each other, especially those of other races or cultures. What a dear thought and expression to share with a friend!

LAUGHTER

Laughter is great medicine. A quiet unassuming young patient, Evelyn had always wanted a tattoo but was not sure she really dared have one because they become permanent on day one. When she lost her hair during chemo, she decided the time was appropriate and so was the place – right on the back of her bald scalp. She found a tattoo artist who drew a cartoon of Betty Boop, a comic strip character whom Evelyn had enjoyed during her childhood. Evelyn told people, "Anything for a chuckle!" For shy Evelyn, the tattoo represented her secret desire to become a carefree outgoing young lady. Unlike most tattoos, the colors were vivid the entire time the design was visible. By the time Betty Boop's scale turned purple, Evelyn's hair had covered her head once more. For this mild-mannered woman, it had served its purpose of allowing her to keep her sense of humor intact. It also fulfilled a whim that had become a challenge to her. Today Evelyn is a gently-assertive woman.

MAÑANA

Ada, a young Mexican woman, was the housekeeper for a couple whose young son Jimmy was undergoing chemotherapy. He always tried very hard to be brave but needed the tender loving care offered by his family and also by Ada. Usually Jimmy readily cheered up as he and Ada sang and played together; so when he began feeling better several days after his chemo sessions, they would chant this little ditty:

Sana, sana, colita de rana,
Si no salva hoy, salvara mañana.

Heal, heal, little frog tail,
If it doesn't heal today, it'll heal tomorrow.

MOM'S MEMORY

Having heard how memory often is adversely affected by anesthesia and chemo, David came to check on his mother-in-law's current status following her surgery and first treatment. He announced his presence inside the house in the family's traditional way by calling out, "Mom, are you here now?" The response was a very clear, "Yes." Then she added, "So far I think I'm here both mentally and physically. Come on in and tell me if I'm right!"

MOTHER & DAUGHTER

Lori and her mother had cancer treatments around the same time. Lori's surgery was in her left breast while her mother's was in her right breast. Lori's comment made both of them laugh when she stated, "Now when we embrace, we'll blend together like a jigsaw puzzle!"

MYSTERY

While living in the Hope Lodge community, Maggie took clothes to the communal laundry room where eight washers and dryers were used by the residents. Since she planned to go shopping that morning, she arose early to start her laundry before drinking her coffee. After finishing breakfast, she ambled over to fold the clothes before leaving. They were not in any of the dryers! Calling it the mystery of the day, she announced to all residents still around the breakfast tables that her clothes were missing and requested that whoever discovered clothes that wouldn't fit could just leave them on the laundry room table. When Maggie returned later, a friend said that the mystery was solved and showed Maggie her neatly folded clothes. All was innocent enough, but for days Maggie blushed and chuckled, repeatedly having to admit that she had simply neglected to transfer anything from the washing machine! She should have blamed it on her *chemobrain* since everyone else uses that excuse.

"NO" TO AN I.D.

Lil was extremely nauseated a couple nights after her first chemo session. She vomited so long that by midnight she and her husband were frightened. She became weaker and more dehydrated. Eddie phoned their doctor.

> *Eddie:* Sorry it's so late, but Lil is as weak as a kitten and has been vomiting for hours. She can't quit for more than 20 minutes. Can you prescribe anything I can get for her tonight?
>
> *Doc:* I'll call your all-night pharmacy right away. They'll have some anti-nausea suppositories that should help.
>
> *Eddie:* Gee, thanks. Lil is too weak to go with me. Do you think I should take her I.D. along with me to get it?
>
> *Doc:* Look, Eddie, these suppositories aren't a controlled substance and I honestly don't believe they will ever catch on as a recreational drug! Good luck and good night.

NORTH CAROLINA DECISION

In 2003 Mary and George were spending the first months of summer in a leased North Carolina cabin when a routine visit to her family doctor turned out to be a diagnosis of breast cancer. Returning at once to their Florida hometown for treatment, she underwent surgery and spent the ensuing months taking chemo. Mary was midway through the treatments when it was time to decide whether or not to renew their lease for the next year. They had no idea how ill she might be the following summer. At the same time, they realized that the anticipation of a return would give them a focal point on which to concentrate their positive hopes of her being able to spend her recovery in their vacation home. Mary was concerned about the cost of their committing themselves to a full summer in case they were unable to return. George squelched her fears with one exceptional remark. He said, "Don't worry, honey; I've already set aside money for the cabin and if we don't get to return, we'll just pretend that we did!" Yes, the following year they were in their favorite retreat in time to see the blooming of the daffodils and the dogwood trees!

RELAY FOR LIFE

At a Relay for Life sponsored by the American Cancer Society, Kay, a breast cancer patient who had just recently entered her recovery stage, was enlightened when she and her husband overheard two survivors walking and talking together. The first said to her partner, "No matter what any doctors say, it took me over a year to overcome the side effects of chemo and radiation." The second survivor replied, "It did for me too; though it was relatively easy compared to the treatments themselves. It really took me months longer than I had expected. If I had only known at the start that recovery would be so gradual, I would've been better prepared." Bill and Kay both thought Kay's recovery was much too gradual to be normal. When they heard this conversation, they grinned and slowed their pace in order to speak freely to each other. They agreed that both had believed Kay might even be regressing because her progress seemed so unpredictable and erratic. Now both understand that the true lesson taught by recovery is patience, patience, patience!

SAINT PATRICK'S DAY

Janice's son Dan came home from college for the weekend to check on his mother's health and enjoy a nice Irish home-cooked meal. It happened to be March 17th and she was feeling well enough to make a green salad for him with green Jell-O on the side. He approached her for a warm motherly hug, laughing and saying, "Gee, Mom, it's a good thing you have cancer; if you didn't, I'd have to pinch you since it's St. Paddy's Day and you aren't wearing the green!" Putting a large lettuce leaf on top of her wig, Janice smiled and said, "Well, now I'm safe from pinches by anyone else!"

SKINNY EYEBROWS

Upon seeing that her Granny's eyebrows were literally only one hair thick, one of Portia's grandchildren said, "Wow, Grandma! With those skinny eyebrows, you look like a super model!"

SO MANY QUESTIONS

Everyone with questions between appointments has probably been urged by physicians to call the office. One of the nurses can often set your mind at ease or have the doctor call you at the end of the workday. Not wanting to be a pest after quizzing the same friendly nurse several times in two days, Lila had yet another question. When she mentioned how much she hated to call again so soon, her grandson gave her a big grin and said, "Oh yeah, I'm sure that nice nurse really hates her job and will say, 'Oh, that silly ole worried woman with breast cancer is such a pain in the neck!' Just call, Grandma." Lila laughed along with her grandson as she reached for the telephone.

TEDDY BEAR HAIR

After Woodi had lost her hair during chemo, she was eagerly expecting her young grandchild to accompany her son and daughter-in-law for a visit. Woodi was worried about the reaction of a three-year old, fearing that Sean might be frightened when his grandma looked so strangely different. Since Woodi still had a bit of soft fuzzy hair, she prepared Sean by suggesting that he bring his teddy bear along. When Sean agreed, Woodi laughingly replied, "Good, you'll be able to feel your teddy bear and then my soft 'teddy bear hair.'" The situation became more fun for both grandmother and grandson as later visits found Woodi with more soft curly hair growing in while the toy teddy's hair remained short and straight.

TELEMARKETER

It happened that a telemarketer named Emily phoned a housewife we'll call Louise. Emily was asking for donations to help buy tombstones for indigent families who could afford only the funeral itself. Louise responded, "Sorry, not this year. I am recovering from breast cancer so all of our family contributions this time are going to the American Cancer Society." The telemarketer sympathized, "I truly understand. The ACS helped finance my own breast cancer treatments just two years ago." The two women talked for some time about the importance of faith and attitude. Then Emily said, "Best of luck to you, Louise," but closed the conversation by adding, "So next year when you are well again, I'm sure you'll give a donation to help some family whose loved one *didn't* survive!" I guess no one could respond negatively to that!

THIMBLE

Unable to sleep well on the eve of her birthday, Elizabeth yearned for the company of her mother who had died a few months earlier. She was feeling especially blue that night because she was soon scheduled to begin radiation treatments, and she yearned for her mother's warm comfort and sound advice during her ongoing battle. Browsing in her bookcase to try to redirect her mood, Elizabeth was surprised to come upon an empty padded envelope. It was one that her mother had kept on hand for special occasions whenever she sent a new thimble for Elizabeth's large collection. Fingering the small package, she felt in close contact with her mother. She shed joyful tears as she turned it over to enjoy her mother's graceful handwriting and then wept openly. Right beside the address her mother had written "Happy Birthday."

TONIGHT'S WIG CHOICE

Blonde jokes abound in every section of our country because lovely beauties are cruelly mistaken, perhaps through the jealousy of others, for possessing less than standard brain power. With that in mind, you will be able to understand Connie's tale. As a temporarily bald chemo patient, she possessed a variety of wigs – blonde, brunette, gray, and silver. For a special dinner party with about 20 friends, Connie looked fabulous in her choice of a blonde wig for the night. During the evening, Connie made a few silly errors in judgment and in speech, all noted by her bevy of friends. They told her not to worry about any imperfections and just giggle along with the crowd. Then one of them teasingly added, "Yeah, you play the blonde role perfectly." Connie's response was to snatch off her wig exposing her baldness and say, "Actually, I'm an intellectual pretending to be a regular member of this group."

Chapter 16

Monthly Medical Records

A sample form for keeping records of
deductible expenditures not covered
by your insurance

Deductibles Not Covered By Insurance:

+ Cash paid
+ Checks
+ Credit cards
+ Mileage
+ Purchased items, etc.

Under existing circumstances, even if Medicare is the
primary insurance in place, many other medically-
related costs incurred include items eligible for
consideration when income tax time comes. Keeping
a current record can be of inestimable value for you
and/or your tax consultant. Perhaps your caregiver
will be willing to help you keep track of many or
all expenses, thereby relieving you of accounting
concerns. Here is a sample form that you may want
to alter for your own use.

Date	Mileage or Item	Amount

Bibliography

1. Book :

Merriam-Webster's *New World Medical Dictionary, Second Edition,* Wiley Publishing, Inc., 909 Third Avenue, New York, NY 10022

2. Booklets and Newsletters :

American Cancer Society (ACS) :

After Diagnosis : 4, 11, 13, 15-16, 25, 27, 35-36

Breast Cancer Update, Issue One 2002: 1-8

Listen With Your Heart : 4, 8-10

Living Smart : 3-4, 12

Sexuality & Cancer : 15, 22-24, 38

National Cancer Institute (NCI)

Eating Hints For Cancer Patients: 17-25, 29-38

Radiation Therapy And You 3, 5-7, 11, 13, 16, 25, 30, 34-44

Understanding Breast Cancer Treatment: 59-66

What You Need To Know About Breast Cancer: 42-50

3. Handout Sheets :

Martin Memorial Cancer Center, Stuart, FL, handout on nutritional services for weight gain or maintenances containing many recipes and nutritious suggestions.

Shands Cancer Center at the University of Florida, Gainesville, FL, publication entitled "Food and Nutritional Services."

4. Pamphlets :

American Cancer Society
After Diagnosis
Listen With Your Heart.
Living Smart.
Services For Patients And Families.
Winn-Dixie Hope Lodge, University of Florida, Gainesville.

National Cancer Institute
Eating Hints For Cancer Patients.
Radiation Therapy And You.
Understanding Breast Cancer Treatments.

5. Personal experiences of other breast cancer patients and my own.

ACKNOWLEDGEMENTS

More thanks than I know how to express go to the kind people who supported me during my battle with breast cancer. Your prayers and concerns uplifted me and made me stronger physically, mentally, and spiritually.

Each of you provided the initial inspiration for this book. Of course special thanks go to editor George Scott of Fountain City Publishing Company, without whom no one would be able to read this information about cancer's side effects and hopes for the future. As I gathered material and ideas toward this publication, my heartfelt gratitude was extended to so many.

All of my cancer health care teams for their excellent care:

Dr. Paul Gaeta, my primary doctor, Martin Memorial Diagnostic Center in Stuart, FL, for his unhurried health care, counseling, and immediate manuscript advice;

Dr. Daniel Dennison, my chemotherapy oncologist, and his staff at Stuart Oncology Associates in Stuart, FL, for curative treatments, sensitive understanding, and donated-entry ideas for this book;

Shands Hospital's Dr. Edward Copeland, my surgeon; Dr. Barbara Shea, my hemotherapist; Dr. Nancy Mendenhall, my radiology oncologist, and all of their terrific staffs at both Shands and the Cancer Center in Gainesville, FL.

Devoted friends for their loving kindnesses to Bill and me:

Dr. Pam Reiner Sandow, longtime friend and member of the University of Florida faculty in the College of Dentistry, who at Shands treated my husband and me like family during my surgery and radiation treatments, as well as during each of my follow-up visits;

Dr. Suzanne Hoekstra of Brevard, NC, who diagnosed my tumor as malignant, and Dr. Margaret Palmer Ayres, lifelong friend of Ocala, FL, both of whom reviewed early drafts of this book for medical accuracy;

Louise Harford and Phyllis Wood, close friends who separately inspected my early manuscript for comprehension and quality;

Janice Howard, my dear friend for 40 years, who drove me places on many Saturdays during my cancer recovery period and, at the end of preparing this book, was my final details-checker.

Connie Bondelid, fellow teacher and artist friend, who perfected my logo design exactly to my specifications;

Nancy M. Copple, friend, Jell-O maker, and fellow language-lover, who critiqued this book and then cheerfully wrote its foreword;

Diane Ebling, computer-savvy friend, who came to my rescue every time I called for help because of my limited PC skills;

My Eta Delta chapter of Chi Omega and my CI chapter of P.E.O. sisters, who showered me with their love and warmth in various unexpected ways;

Sylvia Blee, a P.E.O. sister in Chapter BT, who introduced me to two of Asheville's American Cancer Society representatives with their inside knowledge and encouraging words;

Nancy Smythe, who contributed several hints from her own cancer experiences along with the anecdote about a woman named Hope;

George W. B. Scott, our son, and R. Gideon Scott, our grandson, both of whom helped print my logo and solve some computer glitches by methods unknown to me;

In Stuart: Dr. James Bailey II and our Peace Presbyterian Church family. Jim is totally unaware of the ways that he continues to encourage and enlighten my spirit.

In Brevard, NC:

Pastor Don Waters and his wife Joan from Carson's Creek Baptist Church, along with special friends there including Ada and Dale Crane, Todd Waters, James and Becky Owen, Maurice Cassell, Marjorie Hardin, and songstress Donna Hall. Other church members also offered us support through their prayers.

Margaret J. Scott, friend, writer, and sister-in-law, who offered suggestions and welcome comments during my final editing process.

Dear friends too numerous to mention, dozens of gracious acquaintances, physicians, and nurses who kept me focused by their encouragement and advice during my health treatments and the writing of this book.

Thanks to all our precious supportive children, each of whom visited their father and me during my treatment days and journal writings that became the basis for this book:

Nancy Scott Millar, who flew from Texas to drive us to Shands. She later E-mailed suggestions and several personal stories from her experiences when she, too, underwent breast cancer treatments a few months after mine;

Loring Scott Freeman, who came from Ohio and also drove us to Gainesville. On another visit she mentioned particular topics that needed to be included in my text;

George & Mary Leidig Scott, Portia & Troy A. McDonald, Michael & Amy Scott Schlafer, all of whom offered suggestions along with periodic computer and editing advice.

Chief among my supporters during the "bad days" were William R. "Bill" Scott, my beloved husband; Portia Scott McDonald, my devoted daughter; and Nancy Bracken Fuller, my dear sister:

—Bill was my in-house caregiver during all my treatments and drove me to them. He became my major sounding board while I was writing this book. He was always willing and able to advise me wisely, to critique my thoughts and cheer my efforts, to withstand my lengthy withdrawals into my den, and to prepare countless meals so that I would not be interrupted. In addition, his temperament was, as always, exemplary.

—Portia was my only local offspring during my cancer treatments, although Elizabeth Dennis was nearby and checked on me often. Attorney Portia took care of my legal needs regarding this book, but more personally significant, she was my on-the-spot mainstay. She spent numerous hours nursing me during my side effects and, by her presence, brought great comfort to her father as well.

—Sister Nancy gave me the gift of her advice and organizational talents, along with donating hours upon hours of her time to proofing. I'm sure that "Only If…" would have been a substandard endeavor without her help and persistent attempts for perfection. Actually, she was as obsessed with the exactness of word selection and placement as I was myself.

Finally, extra special thanks to the superb staff and my fellow patients-in-treatment at ACS's Winn-Dixie Hope Lodge in Gainesville. I feel truly blessed to have been associated with each of you and wish you well.

CBS

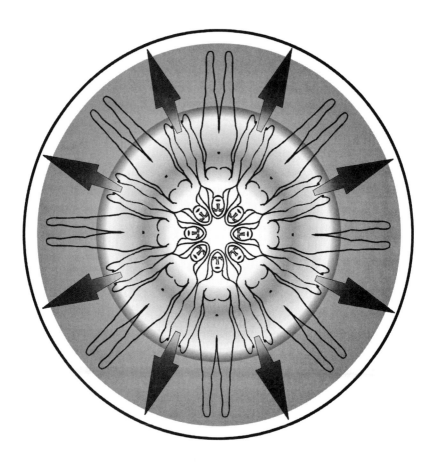

Index

A

B

C

K

S

T

U

V

W

PERSONAL NOTES

_____

_____

_____

_____

_____

_____

_____

_____

PERSONAL NOTES

PERSONAL NOTES

PERSONAL NOTES

_____

_____

_____

_____

_____

_____

_____

_____

PERSONAL NOTES

_____

_____

_____

_____

_____

_____

_____

_____

PERSONAL NOTES

NOTES ABOUT THE AUTHOR

Catharine Bracken Scott was born in Ocala, Florida. She graduated from Salem Academy in North Carolina and earned her degree from Stephens College in Missouri before becoming one of the first full-time coeds to attend the University of Florida. She married William R. Scott in 1950. The following year, she joined *The Ocala Star Banner* staff as society editor. Next they moved south to Stuart and reared five children. During that time Catharine returned to the classroom as a student, commuting to Florida Atlantic University, for her B.A. and M.Ed. degrees.

She taught high school English in the Martin County School System. Later she was an adjunct instructor at both the Stuart branch of Indian River Community College and a local branch of Florida Institute of Technology. Catharine subsequently established her own tutorial school. Called *Conversations with Casey*, its main goal was to motivate students while helping them with their classroom problems.

All of Catharine's writings are non-fiction. In addition to the book in hand, they include *Dear Children*, *Character Sketches*, and *Golden Sparks*, plus *What is this Weird Thing?* (a current manuscript).

Catharine's life in retirement has been devoted to writing books and inventing educational games, although she always takes time to enjoy her large group of treasured friends and deeply-loved family members.

Copies of
Only If You Really Want To Know
are available from:

Therapeia Biblion
P. O. Box 18477
Knoxville, TN   37928

or online at:

www. FCPub.com/Therapeia

Cost per book: $9.95

(Add $.92 per book if ordering
from Tennessee)

$2.50 S&H for first book,
$.50 for each additional book

Please contact us at the above address about special
pricing for libraries and health related facilities